Acamprosate in Relapse Prevention of Alcoholism

Springer
Berlin
Heidelberg
New York
Barcelona
Budapest
Hong Kong
London
Milan
Paris
Santa Clara
Singapore
Tokyo

M. Soyka (Ed.)

Acamprosate in Relapse Prevention of Alcoholism

With 47 Figures and 16 Tables

Springer

PD Dr. Michael Soyka
Psychiatrische Klinik und Poliklinik
der Universität München
Nußbaumstr. 7
80336 München, Germany

ISBN-13:978-3-642-80195-2 e-ISBN-13:978-3-642-80193-8
DOI: 10.1007/978-3-642-80193-8

Library of Congress Cataloging-in-Publication Data. Acamprosate in relapse prevention of alcoholism/ M.Soyka, ed. p. cm. Includes bibliographical references and index. ISBN-13:978-3-642-80195-2 (hardcover)1. Alcoholism - Chemotherapy. 2. Acamprosate. 3. Alcoholism - Relapse - Chemoprevention. I. Soyka. M. (Michael). 1959- . RC565.A27 1996 96-12923

Softcover reprint of the hardcover 1st edition 1996

Cover design: Design & Production, Heidelberg

Typesetting: Scientific Publishing Services (P) Ltd, Madras

SPIN: 10525036 25/3134/SPS - 5 4 3 2 1 0 - Printed on acid-free paper

Preface

Alcoholism is the most common psychiatric disorder in most developed countries and a large number of developing countries, as numerous epidemiological and clinical studies have demonstrated. Alcoholism affects the patient's life in many ways and may induce various medical and psychiatric sequelae. Over the past few decades, there have been continued efforts to improve the treatment of alcoholics. Thus different psychotherapeutic approaches have been designed and applied to alcohol treatment. Follow-up studies have demonstrated alcohol treatment to be efficient, with a significant number of patients remaining abstinent. Still, even after long-term inpatient treatment, more than 50% of the patients relapse.

Relapse prevention remains a major challenge in the treatment of alcoholism. Various forms of relapse prevention including group therapy, individual psychotherapy with supportive or behavioral therapy, contingency contracting, and self-help groups have been advocated. All seem to be helpful in some cases and unsuccessful in a significant number of others.

Apart from chemical aversion therapy, various psychopharmacological interventions have been tried for relapse prevention, all with limited or no success. In recent years, our knowledge of the neurochemical and neurobiological basis of alcoholism and craving for alcohol has increased significantly. The glutamatergic system has been a major focus, and acamprosate, a modulator of the glutamatergic system, is one of the most promising new pharmacological agents used in relapse prevention of alcoholism. In September 1995, a satellite symposium was held prior to the ESBRA congress to evaluate and discuss preclinical and clinical studies conducted with acamprosate. The proceedings of this symposium are summarized in this book, which also contains some important new papers on the pharmacology and clinical efficacy of acamprosate. The editor feels that this book offers a comprehensive overview on the most important studies on acamprosate conducted so far. It is hoped that many patients will benefit from anticraving drugs such as acamprosate, and perhaps this agent will help improve the treatment outcome in alcoholic patients.

Munich
February 1996

Michael Soyka

Contents

List of Contributors

al Qatari, M., Pharmacology Group, Kings College, Manresa Road, London SW3 6LX, UK

Aubin, H.-J., Centre d'Alcoologie, Hôpital Emile Roux, 94456 Limeil-Brévannes Cedex, France

Bottlender, R., Psychiatrische Klinik der Ludwig-Maximilians-Universität, Nußbaumstr. 7, 80336 München, Germany

Chabac, S., Groupe LIPHA, DiMI, 34 rue St-Romain, 69379 Lyon Cedex 8, France

Dahchour, A., Laboratoire de Psychobiologie, Université de Louvain, Place Croix-du-Sud, 1348 Louvain-la-Neuve, Belgium

De Witte, P., Laboratoire de Psychobiologie, Université de Louvain, Place Croix-du-Sud, 1348 Louvain-la-Neuve, Belgium

Durbin, P., Groupe LIPHA, Centre de Recherche et de Développement, 115 avenue Lacassagne, 69003 Lyon, France

Gallinat, J., Psychiatrische Klinik der Ludwig-Maximillians-Universität, Nußbaumstr. 7, 80336 München, Germany

Gillet, C., Centre d'Alcoologie, Hôpital Fournier, 36 quai de la Bataille, 54035 Nancy Cedex, France

Hauser, C., Max-Planck-Institut für Psychiatrie, Klinisches Institut, Kraepelinstr. 2, 80804 München, Germany

Hegerl, U., Psychiatrische Klinik der Ludwig-Maximilians-Universität, Nußbaumstr. 7, 80336 München, Germany

Hulot, T., Groupe LIPHA, Centre de Recherche et de Développement, 115 avenue Lacassagne, 69003 Lyon, France

Kathmann, N., Psychiatrische Klinik der Ludwig-Maximilians-Universität, Nußbaumstr. 7, 80336 München, Germany

Le Bon, O., Laboratoire de Psychobiologie Medicale et d'Alcoologie, Université Libre de Bruxelles (Campus Brugmann), Place Van Gehuchten 4, 1020 Brussels, Belgium

Lehert, P., Département de Sciences Economiques Appliquées, Facultés Catholiques de Mons, 7000 Mons, Belgium

Little, H., Psychology Department, University of Durham, Durham, UK

Littleton, J., Pharmacology Group, Kings College, Manresa Road, London SW3 6LX, UK

Lovinger, D.M., Department of Molecular Physiology and Biophysics and Pharmacology, Vanderbilt University School of Medicine, Nashville, TN 37232-0615, USA

Möller, H.-J., Psychiatrische Klinik der Ludwig-Maximilians-Universität, Nußbaumstr. 7, 80336 München, Germany

Paille, F., Centre d'Alcoologie, Hôpital Fournier, 36 quai de la Bataille, 54035 Nancy Cedex, France

Parot, P., Pharmaceutical Consultant, 12, avenue G. Pompidon, 92800 Puteaux, France

Pelc, I., Laboratoire de Psychologie Medicale et d'Alcoologie, Université Libre de Bruxelles (Campus Brugmann), Place Van Gehuchten 4, 1020 Brussels, Belgium

Potgieter, A.S., Groupe LIPHA, 34 rue St-Romain, 69379 Lyon Cedex 8, France

Preuß, U., Psychiatrische Klinik der Ludwig-Maximilians-Universität, Nußbaumstr. 7, 80336 München, Germany

Putzke, J., Max-Planck-Institut für Psychiatrie, Klinisches Institut, Kraepelinstr. 2, 80804 München, Germany

Quertemont, E., Laboratoire de Psychobiologie, Université de Louvain, Place Croix-du-Sud, 1348 Louvain-la-Neuve, Belgium

Siggins, G.R., Department of Neuropharmacology, The Scripps Research Institute, 10666 North Torrey Pines Road, La Jolla, CA 92037, USA

Soyka, M., Psychiatrische Klinik der Ludwig-Maximilians-Universität, Nußbaumstr. 7, 80336 München, Germany

Spanagel, R., Max-Planck-Institut Für Psychiatrie, Klinisches Institut, Kraepelinstr. 2., 80804 München, Germany

Ufer, S., Psychiatrische Klinik der Ludwig-Maximilians-Universität, Nußbaumstr. 7, 80336 München, Germany

Verbanck, P., Laboratoire de Psychologie Medicale et d'Alcoologie, Université Libre de Bruxelles (Campus Brugmann), Place Van Gehuchten 4, 1020 Brussels, Belgium

Wetzel, C., Max-Planck-Institut für Psychiatrie, Klinisches Institut, Kraepelinstr. 2, 80804 München, Germany

Zieglgänsberger, W., Max-Planck-Institut für Psychiatrie, Klinisches Institut, Kraepelinstr. 2, 80804 München, Germany

Ethanol and the NMDA Receptor: Implications for Intoxication, Tolerance, Dependence, and Alcoholic Brain Damage

D.M. Lovinger

Introduction

Most alcohol users take for granted the effects of the drug on movement, memory as well as the anxiolytic effects often experienced upon ingestion of moderate amounts of alcoholic drinks. In addition, the majority of persons are well aware of the existence of alcoholism and hence of the fact that alcohol is addictive. It is also widely known that use of the drug over a long timespan leads to brain damage. Despite this widespread knowledge of alcohol's actions we are just beginning to appreciate the neural actions of alcohol which lead to these outcomes.

Ethanol (EtOH) produces all of the aforementioned actions primarily through effects on the central nervous system, and actions on the brain in particular (see Koob and Bloom 1988; Dietrich et al. 1989; Koob 1992). Recent research efforts have been directed at understanding the way in which EtOH alters the function of brain circuitry, individual neurons and molecules important for neuronal function (see Koob and Bloom 1988; Shefner 1990; Samson and Harris 1992; Sanna and Harris 1993 for review). What is emerging is a picture of acute EtOH effects beginning with actions at specific molecular targets leading to alterations in neuronal activity. Ultimately, behavior is altered as a consequence of these neural changes.

The effects of chronic EtOH exposure appear to arise from changes in the CNS that compensate for the acute actions of the drug (Buck and Harris 1991; Samson and Harris 1992; Lovinger 1993; Tabakoff and Hoffman 1995) and more gradual changes which may have little impact during acute intoxication but accumulate with repeated alcohol exposure (e.g. nutritional changes such as thiamine deficiency; Butterworth et al. 1993; Charness 1993; Manzo et al. 1994). The compensatory changes involve many of the same molecules that are affected by acute EtOH exposure (Allan and Harris 1987; Dolin et al. 1987; Greenberg et al. 1987; Skattebol and Rabin 1987; Morrow et al. 1988; Grant et al. 1990b; Buck and Harris 1991; Gulya et al. 1991; Montpied et al. 1991; Dildy-Mayfield and Harris 1992a; Hoffman et al. 1992; Iorio et al. 1992; Lovinger 1993; Mhatre and Ticku 1993; Trevisan et al. 1994; Tabakoff and Hoffman 1995). These changes may act cooperatively with other factors to induce undesirable

Departments of Molecular Physiology and Biophysics and Pharmacology, Vanderbilt University School of Medicine, Nashville, TN 37232-0615, USA consequences of chronic EtOH abuse such as alcohol dependence and brain damage.

The molecular targets of acute EtOH action are just beginning to come into focus. Among the neuromolecules thought to be involved in intoxication are neurotransmitter receptors including those activated by GABA, glutamate, serotonin and acetylcholine, voltage-gated calcium channels, neurotransmitter transporters and certain enzymes involved in intracellular signaling (Shefner 1990; Wang et al. 1991; Samson and Harris 1992; Gordon et al. 1993; Lovinger and Peoples 1993; Miller 1993; Sanna and Harris 1993; Sun et al. 1993; Weight et al. 1993; Tabakoff and Hoffman 1995). This review concentrates on EtOH actions on the *N*-methyl-D-asparate (NMDA) type of glutamate receptor. Literature will be discussed which indicates that this receptor plays an important role in all of the EtOH actions mentioned above.

Glutamate-Activated Ligand-Gated Ion Channels

Glutamate is used as a neurotransmitter at most synapses connecting different regions of the mammalian brain and at many of the synapses involved in local circuit connections within brain regions (see Mayer and Westbrook 1987a; Greenamyre and Porter 1994 for review). Glutamate excites all central neurons in part by activating receptors which contain an intrinsic ion channel (Barnes and Henley 1992; Seeburg 1993; Hollman and Heinemann 1994; Nakanishi 1994; Westbrook 1994). These receptors, members of a receptor family known as the ligand-gated ion channels, allow cations to pass from the outside to the inside of neurons, creating inward currents which depolarize neurons. This depolarization leads neurons to fire action potentials and hence to communicate information to other neurons in a neuronal circuit.

The glutamate-activated ligand-gated ion channels (or ionotropic glutamate receptors) have been subdivided into three groups, the NMDA, kainate. and AMPA receptors, based on their molecular structures and pharmacology (Nakanishi 1994; Hollman and Heinemann 1994; Schoepfer et al. 1994; Westbrook 1994). Each group is named for an agonist which strongly activates that group of receptors. Antagonists have also been developed which preferentially block different receptor types. The amino acid sequence of these receptors has recently been elucidated. It appears that these receptors are formed from the confluence of different subunit proteins as is the case for other ligand-gated ion channels. Several subunits that contribute to the formation of each type of receptor group have been identified. Thus, numerous receptor subtypes may exist within each glutamate receptor group due to the confluence of different subunit combinations.

The different groups of glutamate-activated ligand-gated ion channels also have different functional properties. The NMDA-type receptors are characterized by high calcium permeability and slow channel kinetics (MacDermott et al. 1986; Mayer and Westbrook 1987; Mayer et al. 1987; Jahr and Stevens 1993; Monyer et al. 1994). These receptor/channels remain active for relatively long periods after initial activation and can allow substantial calcium influx during activation. The calcium influx can lead, in turn, to activation of intracellular signaling pathways. The AMPA and kainate receptors have faster channel kinetics and only selected subtypes of these receptors are calcium permeable (Keinanen et al. 1990; Verdoorn et al. 1991; Jonas and Spruston 1994). These receptors are involved in fast electrical signaling at glutamatergic synapses. NMDA receptors are thought to participate in initiation of synaptic plasticity both during development of the CNS and in adult animals (Morris et al. 1986; Collingridge and Bliss 1987; Hestrin 1992; Carmignoto and Vicini 1992; Komuro and Rakic 1993). Long-term potentiation (LTP) of synapses in the hippocampus is the best characterized example of a plastic change in synaptic efficacy involving NMDA receptor activation (Collingridge and Bliss 1987). NMDA receptors may also participate in synaptic development (Dow and Riopelle 1990; Carmignoto and Vicini 1992; Komuro and Rakic 1993). The AMPA receptors are the workhorses of excitatory synaptic transmission in the CNS. These receptors provide the bulk of fast synaptic excitation at CNS glutamatergic synapses, providing electrical excitation that is necessary for communication of information both within and between brain regions (c.f. MacDermott and Dale 1987; Mayer and Westbrook 1987a; Andreasen et al. 1989). However, these receptors may also play a crucial role in initiating plastic synaptic events in brain regions such as the cerebellum (Linden 1994).

Acute EtOH Exposure Inhibits the Function of NMDA and Other Glutamate Receptors

As the reader can probably surmise from the foregoing discussion, alteration of the function of ionotropic glutamate receptors would likely have a profound impact on brain and behavior. Thus, it is important to determine the actions of EtOH on these receptors and on synaptic transmission at glutamatergic synapses. Early studies of acute EtOH effects on excitatory, glutamatergic synaptic transmission in brain slices indicated only small effects of the drug on fast excitatory postsynaptic potentials (EPSPs; Rogers et al. 1979; Siggins et al. 1987; Lovinger et al. 1990). EtOH did, however, interfere with the initiation of LTP in the CA1 region of the hippocampus (Sinclair and Lo 1986; Mulkeen et al. 1987; Blitzer et al. 1990; Morrisett and Swartzwelder 1993). We now know that the fast EPSPs examined in these earlier studies are mediated predominantly by activation of AMPA or kainate receptors while initiation of LTP involves activation of NMDA receptors. Thus, studies of glutamatergic transmission indicated that EtOH might be a more potent inhibitor of transmission mediated by NMDA than by non-NMDA ionotropic glutamate receptors. This finding has been confirmed in more recent studies indicating that EtOH inhibits pharmacologically isolated NMDA receptor-mediated EPSPs in hippocampus more potently than it inhibits EPSPs mediated by non-NMDA receptors (Lovinger et al. 1990; Morrisett et al. 1991; Grover et al. 1994).

A more direct demonstration of EtOH effects on receptor function was provided by studies examining the effects of EtOH on glutamate receptor function in more isolated neuronal preparations. In these experiments receptors were activated by direct agonist application to intact neurons, and receptor function was assayed by measuring ion current, calcium influx, or stimulated neurotransmitter secretion. The findings from these experiments generally supported the idea that EtOH inhibits NMDA receptors at pharmacologically relevant concentrations (5–100 mM) in a variety of neuronal preparations including brain slices and cultured and acutely isolated neurons (Dildy and Leslie 1989; Göthert and Fink 1989; Hoffman et al 1989a; Lima-Landman and Albuquerque 1989; Lovinger et al. 1989; Woodward and Gonzales 1990). EtOH appears to be less potent in inhibiting the function of non-NMDA ionotropic glutamate receptors (Hoffman et al. 1989a; Lovinger et al. 1989). Recent studies of non-NMDA receptors expressed in heterologous expression systems such as *Xenopus* oocytes and human embryonic kidney cells indicate that some AMPA receptors exhibit EtOH sensitivity higher than observed in past studies of neurons (Dildy-Mayfield and Harris 1992a,b; Lovinger 1993). These studies suggest that EtOH effects on some subtypes of these receptors may occur at more physiologically relevant concentrations. However, at present there is little information from neuronal preparations to support this idea. Thus, this discussion concentrates on EtOH actions on the NMDA receptor.

Table 1 summarizes the current state of knowledge about the mechanism of acute EtOH actions on the NMDA receptor. It is worth noting that EtOH acts within milliseconds to inhibit receptor function and inhibition is fully reversible over a time course consistent with removal of EtOH from a given preparation (Lovinger and Peoples 1993). Thus, the effect appears to depend on the continued presence of EtOH and is not a consequence of activation of a long-lasting change in cellular or channel properties.

Table 1. Characteristics of acute EtOH inhibition of NMDA receptors

Inhibition is rapid and reversible	Lovinger et al. 1989; Lovinger and Peoples 1993
EtOH inhibits single NMDA-activated channels	Lima-Landman and Albuquerque 1989; Weight et al. 1993
Potency of alcohols increases with increasing hydrophobicity	Lovinger et al. 1989; Fink and Göthert 1990; Gonzales et al. 1991; Peoples and Weight 1995
No effect on desensitization	Lovinger and Peoples 1993
Inhibition is not use, or voltage dependent, EtOH is not a channel blocker	Weight et al. 1993
Noncompetitive with NMDA	Hoffman et al. 1989b; Woodward and Gonzales 1990; Dildy-Mayfield and Leslie 1991; Weight et al. 1993
Glycine Reversal of Inhibition	Woodward and Gonzales 1990; Rabe and Tabakoff 1990; Dildy-Mayfield and Leslie 1991; see also Jones and Leslie 1993; Weaver et al. 1993
Noncompetitive with glycine	Peoples and Weight 1992; Woodward 1994
Noncompetitive with Phencyclidine, polyamine, proton sites on receptor	Hoffman et al. 1989b; Peoples, Lovinger, White and Weight, unpublished observations; Weight et al. 1993
Interactions with Mg^{2+}	Morrisett et al. 1991; Chandler et al. 1994

The NMDA receptor is modulated by endogenous compounds and drugs which have actions at a number of sites believed to be contained within the receptor protein (see Mayer et al. 1989; Watkins and Oliverman 1987; Wong and Kemp 1991; Ishii et al. 1993 for review). The interactions between EtOH and a number of modulatory sites have been investigated (see Table 1 for summary). There is general agreement on the lack of EtOH interactions with several sites on the receptor (e.g. the NMDA/glutamate binding site, the phencyclidine site). However, there is still some disagreement about interactions with the sites of action of glycine and divalent cations (see references in Table 1). Glycine at micromolar concentrations can overcome the actions of EtOH in cerebellar granule cells and striatal slices, and it was suggested that EtOH interacts with the site at which glycine acts as "coagonist" at the NMDA receptor (Woodward and Gonzales 1990; Rabe and Tabakoff 1990). However, subsequent studies have indicated that EtOH does not alter the potency of glycine for acting at this site and that glycine coagonist site antagonists do not reverse the ability of glycine to reduce EtOH effects (Peoples and Weight 1992; Woodward 1994). The glycine/EtOH interaction is thus more complex than a simple competitive interaction and may be brain region specific. The brain regional specificity may, in turn, relate to brain regional expression of different NMDA receptor subtypes which are discussed below. It is also worth noting that EtOH inhibition of receptor function and reversal of this inhibition by glycine may depend on the agonist which is used for receptor activation (Jones and Leslie 1993; Weaver et al. 1993). Evidence for EtOH interactions with divalent cation binding sites comes from studies using rather indirect measures of receptor function (NMDA-induced excitotoxicity and NMDA receptor mediated responses in brain slices; Martin et al. 1991; Morrisett et al. 1991; Chandler et al. 1994). Thus, it is possible that the interaction involves sites other than the NMDA receptor itself.

Evidence of an interaction between EtOH and the noncompetitive NMDA receptor antagonist ifenprodil has been observed (Lovinger 1995). However, ifenprodil does not appear to interact with the same molecular site on the receptor as that which is responsible for ethanol's actions. Rather, ifenprodil appears selectively to inhibit certain NMDA receptor subtypes, and these subtypes may be more sensitive to inhibition by EtOH. This is discussed in more detail in the following section.

As with most targets of alcohol actions, it is not clear whether the primary site of the molecular actions of EtOH which alter NMDA receptors is a lipid or protein. It has been repeatedly demonstrated that the potency of alcohols for inhibiting NMDA receptor function increases with increasing hydrophobicity (Lovinger et al. 1989; Fink and Göthert 1990; Gonzales et al. 1991; Peoples and Weight 1995). However, this relationship may reflect of an interaction with lipids or with hydrophobic portions of a protein. A recent study demonstrated that the relationship between alcohol potency and hydrophobicity breaks down when *n*-alkanols of chain length greater than eight carbons are used (Peoples and Weight 1995). It has been argued that this "cutoff" effect is inconsistent with actions on a lipid bilayer since one would expect lipid perturbation to occur during treatment with the longer chain, more hydrophobic alcohols.

These investigators, following up on the idea put forth by Franks and Lieb (1985), suggest that the cutoff phenomenon is due to the fact that alcohols interact with hydrophobic pockets on proteins and that the size of the pocket associated with the NMDA receptor is such that longer chain alcohols cannot fit. Alternative scenarios in which cutoff can occur even when lipids are involved in an effect have been proposed (Alifimoff et al. 1989; Raines et al. 1993; Wood et al. 1993). A site of alcohol action which is defined by both protein and lipid elements is equally consistent with existing data. Furthermore, it is not clear that all of the alcohols interact at the same single site of action as proposed by proponents of the hydrophobic pocket hypothesis. However, the observation of a cutoff phenomenon does cast doubt on the hypothesis that alcohol alters NMDA receptor function simply by disordering neuronal membranes.

NMDA Receptor Subtypes and Acute Alcohol Actions

Five subunits arising from as many separate genes which can be incorporated into functional NMDA receptors have been discovered and named R1 and R2A–D (Moriyoshi et al. 1991; Kutsuwada et al. 1992; Meguro et al. 1992; Monyer et al. 1992; Ishii et al. 1993). As the names imply, the amino acid sequence of the NMDAR1 subunits is quite distinct from that of the 2A–D subunits. However, there is considerable diversity within the sequences of the four NMDAR2 subunits. In addition, the NMDAR1 gene product can undergo extensive posttranscriptional modification by alternative splicing (Anantharam et al. 1992; Durand et al. 1992; Sugihara et al. 1992). Through a combination of splice sites on both the N- and C-terminal portions of the receptor it is possible to generate NMDAR1 proteins with eight different sequences. A number of subunit combinations can come together to form NMDA receptors. It is suspected that the receptor is formed from the confluence of five subunits. These need not necessarily be five different subunits. Heterologous expression studies indicate that fully functional receptors can be formed by the combination of two different subunits (Kutsuwada et al. 1992; Meguro et al. 1992; Ishii et al. 1993; Monyer et al. 1992, 1994). However, it is suspected that these receptors are pentameric combinations of the constituent subunits.

Recent studies have focused on the relationship between NMDA receptor subunit composition and EtOH sensitivity. The majority of studies have examined acute EtOH actions on NMDA receptors expressed in *Xenopus* oocytes (Koltchine et al. 1993; Buller et al. 1993; Kuner et al. 1993; Masood et al. 1994; Mirshahi and Woodward 1995). This well characterized heterologous expression system allows one to achieve functional expression of neurotransmitter receptors whose function can then be studied using voltage-clamp electrophysiological analysis. Investigators have examined EtOH effects on homomeric NMDA receptors made by the different NMDAR1 splice variants as well as heteromeric receptors which contain combinations of NMDAR1 and different NMDAR2 subunits. Koltchine et al. (1993) reported that EtOH inhibits the function of NMDA receptors made from different NMDAR1 splice variants, and that receptors made with different splice variants exhibit differential sensitivity to EtOH. Interestingly, the high EtOH sensitivity observed in the "long-long" splice variant, which contains inserted "cassettes" at all splice sites, appears to be due to selective inhibition of a long-latency calcium-dependent current seen in receptors containing this variant. Kuner et al. (1993) reported that receptors containing NMDAR1 in combination with NMDAR2A, 2B, or 2C showed approximately equal sensitivity to EtOH. Subsequent studies by Masood et al. (1994), Koltchine et al. (1993), and Mirshahi and Woodward (1995) provide evidence that NMDAR2C-containing receptors or those containing the mouse equivalent have lower EtOH sensitivity than receptors containing NMDAR2A or 2B (or the mouse equivalents). The reason for the difference in the findings of Kuner et al. (1993) and the other investigators is presently unclear. The most prominent methodological difference among the studies is the fact that Kuner et al. (1993) employed glutamate to activate receptors while the other investigators used NMDA. Thus, it is possible that EtOH effects may differ with the agonist used to activate the receptor.

The examination of NMDA receptor function using mammalian heterologous expression systems has also been undertaken. In a recent study Lovinger (1995) examined EtOH effects on recombinant heteromeric NMDA receptors expressed in human embryonic kidney (HEK 293) cells. The results of this analysis resemble the findings of Kuner et al. (1993) in that little difference in EtOH potency was observed among receptors containing NMDAR1A in combination with 2A, 2B, or 2C subunits. However, it was noted that 2A-containing receptors were slightly less sensitive to low concentrations of EtOH.

Another approach to determining the relationship between receptor subunit composition and EtOH sensitivity is to examine native NMDA receptors expressed by neurons. Two approaches have been taken using this strategy. Determining what NMDA receptor subunits are expressed by a given neuron and correlating this information with measures of EtOH sensitivity allows the investigator to rule out involvement of receptors that are not expressed by a given neuron. Work in this area has just begun. Simson et al. (1993) have described brain regional differences in EtOH sensitivity which may be attributable to differences in expression of particular NMDA receptor subunits. However, the measurements of receptor expression are limited to measurements of mRNA expression from groups of cells and thus it is difficult to correlate subunit expression with EtOH sensitivity on a per cell basis. In cultured cortical neurons, EtOH sensitivity of NMDA receptors decreases during the first few weeks of neuronal development (Lovinger 1995), and this decrease coincides with reported changes from predominant NMDAR2B expression to a mixture of 2A and 2B expression (Williams et al. 1993; Zhong et al. 1994). This developmental change in EtOH sensitivity is particularly interesting in that NMDA receptors may participate in neuronal development and potent effects of EtOH on fetal forms of the receptor and may contribute to fetal alcohol effects. Measurements of receptor pharmacology over this developmental period support the idea that receptor subunit composition changes in the majority of neurons, and thus some correlation between receptor changes and EtOH sensitivity has been observed in this preparation (Lovinger 1995).

However, there is little or no information about the expression of the NMDAR1 splice variants and other features of the receptors (e.g. posttranslational modification) at this time. Thus, continued effort is needed to measure receptor subunit expression and protein status in relation to alcohol sensitivity. With the advent of techniques for measuring receptor mRNA expression in single neurons (Eberwine et al. 1992) and the development of subunit-specific antibodies (Sheng et al. 1994) better correlations between subunit expression and EtOH sensitivity should be possible in the near future.

The role of particular NMDA receptor subunits in determining EtOH sensitivity can also be examined using tools which will selectively disrupt the function of particular receptor subtypes. One can compare EtOH sensitivity of NMDA receptors before and after treatment with such agents to determine whether eliminating one receptor subtype alters sensitivity. To date, few selective inhibitors of different receptor subtypes are available. However, the phenylethanolamine ifenprodil selectively inhibits 2B-containing heteromeric receptors (Williams et al. 1993; Williams 1993; Lovinger 1995). Furthermore, treatment with this compound has been shown to reduce EtOH sensitivity of NMDA receptors in cortical neurons that most likely contain a mix of 2A and 2B-containing receptors. This observation suggests that elimination of a subpopulation of 2B-containing receptors removes the most EtOH-sensitive fraction of receptors leaving receptors which are less EtOH-sensitive and presumably contain 2A. However, it is not clear that the presence of NMDAR2B is the sole factor, or even one factor, determining EtOH sensitivity. Since the receptors are presumably complex heteromeric proteins, it is possible that the identity or processing of another subunit which changes along with NMDAR2B participates in determining EtOH sensitivity. Other chemical inhibitors, such as the spider venom derivative argiotoxin 636, have been suggested to have selective effects on NMDA receptors subtypes and may thus be useful in experiments examining EtOH sensitivity (Raditsch et al. 1993). An alternative approach would be to remove particular receptor subunits by antisense oligonucleotide treatment. This would allow investigators selectively to eliminate one receptor subunit and then determine whether EtOH sensitivity is altered.

NMDA Receptor Involvement in EtOH Intoxication

Behavioral studies have examined the question of how EtOH effects on NMDA receptors contribute to acute intoxication. Among the many behavioral changes associated with intoxication are the subjective effects of EtOH, anxiolytic effects, motor impairment, cognitive deficits and general anesthesia (Schuckit 1995; Lovinger and Grant 1995). Administration of NMDA receptor antagonists can produce actions similar to those of EtOH including EtOH-like discriminative stimulus effects, anxiolytic effects and anesthetic effects (Table 2). With regard to the EtOH-like discriminative stimulus effects of NMDA receptor antagonists, interesting recent work suggests that the role of NMDA receptors in ethanol's subjective effects is especially strong in rats trained to recognize the effects of moderate to high EtOH doses (Grant and Colombo 1993a,b).

Table 2. Behavioral evidence for involvement of NMDA receptors in acute EtOH intoxication

Ethanol-like discriminative stimulus effects of NMDA receptor antagonist	Balster et al. 1992; Butelman et al. 1993; Grant et al. 1991; Grant and Colombo 1993a; Sanger 1993
EtOH potentiation of NMDA receptor antagonist anesthetic actions	Boren and Consroe 1981; Fidecka and Langwinski 1989; Wessinger and Balster 1987; Brunet et al. 1986
EtOH Inhibition of LTP and spatial learning/ memory	Steffensen et al. 1993; Criado et al. 1994; Matthews et al. 1995; Devenport and Merriman 1983; Gibson 1985
NMDA receptor antagonists are anxiolytic	Chait et al. 1981; Clineschmidt et al. 1982; Guimares et al. 1991; Liebman and Bennet 1988

Channel blockers appear to substitute better than competitive antagonists with respect to the EtOH interoceptive cue. This may indicate that the mechanism of receptor inhibition is important in determining the subjective effects of the drug.

The involvement of NMDA receptors in EtOH-induced general anesthesia is uncertain. The general anesthesia produced by EtOH does not appear to share characteristics of dissociative anesthesia produced by NMDA receptor/channel blockers (Wong et al. 1986; Lodge et al. 1987; Huettner and Bean 1988; Wong and Kemp 1991) and more closely resembles anesthesia produced by barbiturates or volatile general anesthetics. It is suspected that EtOH-induced anesthesia is mediated by effects on GABAA receptors in the brain. Indeed, the anesthetic effects of barbiturates are potentiated by EtOH (see Dietrich 1987 for review). However, a similar potentiation of the effects of dissociative anesthetics has also been observed (Boren and Consroe 1981; Brunet et al. 1986; Wessinger and Balster 1987; Fidecka and Langwinski 1989). The possibility remains that both GABAA and NMDA receptors participate in EtOH-induced anesthesia, and that changes in drug effects at either receptor alter EtOH potency or efficacy for producing this behavioral effect.

Antagonists at the NMDA receptor have strong inhibitory effects on hippocampal LTP and spatial learning (see Collingridge and Bliss 1987 for review). Thus, it is quite logical to postulate that EtOH inhibition of NMDA receptors contribute to deficits in LTP and cognitive functions involving the hippocampus. Numerous laboratories have reported EtOH inhibition of LTP both in vivo and in brain slices (Sinclair and Lo 1986; Mulkeen et al. 1987; Blitzer et al. 1990; Morrisett and Swartzwelder 1993; Steffensen et al. 1993). The effect of EtOH is on initiation rather than maintenance of LTP, which is similar to the actions of NMDA receptor antagonists. In addition, some studies in hippocampal slices have shown strong links between ethanol inhibition of NMDA receptors and inhibition of LTP (Blitzer et al. 1990; Morrisett and Swartzwelder 1993). However, alternative actions of EtOH that contribute to inhibition of LTP have been suggested. For example, intact projections from the septum or the ventral tegmentum appear to be required for EtOH blockade of LTP in the dentate gyrus in vivo (Steffensen et al. 1993; Criado et al. 1994). This finding suggests that EtOH effects on LTP are indirect in that other brain regions may be the primary sites of EtOH actions. However, it is not clear that removal of the septum does not alter NMDA receptor function in a way that would overcome the incomplete block by EtOH and restore LTP. It is also not clear whether the actions of EtOH on LTP in the CA1 region of brain slices is the same as in the dentate gyrus in vivo. Clearly, more work is needed to clarify the role of NMDA receptors in EtOH blockade of LTP.

Ethanol is known to have actions on performance in learning and memory tasks. The effects of EtOH on state- or context-dependent learning are well known (see Lister 1987 for review). The discovery of EtOH actions on GABAA and NMDA receptors in the hippocampus has led investigators to examine more closely EtOH effects on spatial learning and memory since the function of these receptors in hippocampus is believed to play an important role in these types of learning and memory. It has been reported by several investigators that EtOH impairs spatial memory and working memory (Table II; Matthews et al. 1995; Devenport and Merriman 1983; Gibson 1985). The effect of EtOH on spatial memory is mimicked by MK-801 but not by diazepam, suggesting possible mediation of the EtOH effects by NMDA receptor inhibition (Matthews et al. 1995). In addition to examining EtOH effects on behavioral indices of learning and memory, investigators have focused on determining EtOH effects on neuronal activity related to information storage. This includes studies of EtOH effects on neuronal firing and "theta" frequency EEG activity in neurons of the hippocampus and medial septum. An elegant study by Givens (1995) demonstrated that EtOH reduces choice accuracy on a delayed alternation task in rats at concentrations as low as 0.75 g/kg. Several measures of hippocampal theta activity were recorded in the same rats and EtOH treatment produced reductions in theta prevalence and relative power at concentrations at or below that which altered memory. Recent reports also indicate EtOH inhibition of the firing of spatially related "place cells" in the hippocampus which may play a role in performance of spatial memory tasks (Matthews et al. 1994). It is not yet clear whether these effects of EtOH on neuronal activity are due to NMDA receptor inhibition. Indeed, EtOH-like effects on place cell firing are not observed with either MK-801 or diazepam, indicating the involvement of molecular targets other than or in addition to NMDA and GABAA receptors.

NMDA Receptor Involvement in EtOH Tolerance and Dependence

Two lines of reasoning have led researchers to postulate a role for NMDA receptors in tolerance to EtOH. First, there is strong evidence of a role for NMDA receptors in synaptic plasticity as well as learning and memory (reviewed above) and it is well known that tolerance involves plastic changes in neuronal function and that tolerance can involve a strong learned component (see Grant et al. 1990; Kalant 1993; Tabakoff and Hoffman 1988, 1995). The combination of these ideas stimulated researchers to begin to investigate the role of NMDA receptors in alcohol tolerance (Wu et al. 1993; Khanna et al. 1993; 1994; Szabo et al. 1994). The hypothesis underlying these investigations was that NMDA receptor activation serves as a trigger for synaptic plasticity needed to establish tolerance. NMDA receptor activation might also take place during the learning of contingencies necessary for the development of learned tolerance. Tolerance can be divided into several temporal stages including rapid, acute and chronic stages (Kalant 1993). NMDA receptor antagonists have been shown to block the development of tolerance at all three stages (Wu et al. 1993; Khanna et al. 1993, 1994). However, recent studies suggest that NMDA receptor activation is only necessary for tolerance which has a strong dependence on environmental conditions (Szabo et al. 1994).

The relationship between acute EtOH actions on the NMDA receptor and the role of the receptor in tolerance is unclear. Since EtOH does not completely abolish receptor function at pharmacological concentrations, it is possible that the remaining receptor-mediated activity is sufficient, in combination with other cellular processes, to trigger the mechanisms necessary for initiation of tolerance. Alternatively, it is possible that EtOH inhibition of the receptor decreases with time following initial exposure. This would lead to enhanced NMDA receptor mediated transmission during EtOH exposure which might trigger synaptic plasticity following an initial phase of lessened plasticity. Some support for this hypothesis has been generated in a recent study by Grover et al. (1994). These investigators have observed that EtOH inhibition of NMDA receptor-mediated synaptic transmission decreases over tens of minutes of exposure to EtOH in hippocampal slices. This "acute tolerance" to EtOH might be the trigger for enhanced plasticity that initiates the mechanisms needed for more long-lasting tolerance. However, the question remains as to what mechanisms lead the receptors to show tolerance during acute EtOH exposure. Furthermore, it is not clear that acute tolerance to EtOH effects on NMDA receptors is observed under all conditions (see Lovinger et al. 1990). It is also possible that NMDA receptor function increases following the cessation of EtOH exposure even after one or a few instances of exposure. This could enhance the likelihood of initiating plasticity. There is little evidence at this time regarding the changes in neuronal or synaptic function that underlie NMDA receptor dependent EtOH tolerance. It is tempting to speculate that some process akin to long-term potentiation is involved in this change in neuronal function. However, more direct evidence is needed to support this hypothesis.

NMDA receptors have also been implicated in long-lasting forms of EtOH tolerance. One measure of tolerance to the NMDA receptor-inhibiting effects of EtOH is to examine cross-tolerance between EtOH and other NMDA receptor antagonists. Drugs which have similar effects on a given neurotransmitter receptor often show cross-tolerance in behavioral tests even if the sites of drug actions within the receptor are different. Ethanol tolerant animals exhibit cross-tolerance to MK-801 and competitive NMDA receptor antagonists, at least with certain behavioral measures of tolerance (Danysz et al. 1992). This finding indicates that changes in behavioral pharmacology induced by chronic EtOH exposure involve changes in the function of NMDA receptors in the CNS.

Ethanol tolerance involving the NMDA receptor may arise because the ability of EtOH to inhibit NMDA receptors decreases during chronic EtOH exposure. Alternatively, there may be compensatory changes in the number or function of NMDA receptors which work to counteract the inhibitory effect of acute EtOH exposure. Experiments to date generally support the latter hypothesis. When EtOH inhibition of NMDA receptor function is examined following chronic EtOH exposure the effects of EtOH appear to be unaltered (White et al. 1990; Iorio et al. 1992; Chandler et al. 1993). However, it should be noted that some of these experiments were performed on cells in culture or brain tissue from animals that were not tested for tolerance. Thus, a strong dissociation between tolerance and continued effects of EtOH on the NMDA receptor was not demonstrated.

There is more evidence for changes in the receptor following chronic EtOH exposure. Initial evidence indicated an increase in the number of MK-801 binding sites in hippocampus of tolerant and dependent rats (Valverius et al. 1990; Gulya et al. 1991; Hoffman et al. 1992; Sanna et al. 1993; but see Michaelis et al. 1993; Tremwel et al. 1994). This was taken as evidence for increased numbers of NMDA receptors in this brain region. Other evidence for increased receptor expression has also accumulated, including a recent report of increased expression of NMDAR1 subunit protein in hippocampus after prolonged EtOH treatment (Trevisan et al. 1994). However, the alcohol treatment protocols differ considerably among different laboratories studying this problem. In many of these studies the animals are probably alcohol-dependent as well as tolerant. Thus, the receptor changes may play a larger role in dependence than in tolerance, as discussed in the subsequent section of this review. The methods for measuring receptor number also differ among laboratories, and it is not clear that all of these measures directly reflect numbers of functional receptors. In other studies NMDA receptor function has been examined by measuring receptor-stimulated excitotoxicity, calcium influx, or increases in intracellular calcium in chronic EtOH-treated and control cultured neurons (Iorio et al. 1992, 1993; Chandler et al. 1993; Ahern et al. 1994; Mirshahi et al. 1995; Smothers et al. 1995). These studies generally indicate increased responses to NMDA receptor activation following chronic EtOH exposure. There is some selectively to these changes since responses to activation of non-NMDA receptors are not altered following chronic EtOH exposure (Iorio et al. 1993; Smothers et al. 1995). Behavioral studies in mice indicate that responses to NMDA increase following chronic EtOH exposure (Grant et al. 1990). It is tempting to speculate that these functional changes arise from increases in the number or function of the NMDA receptors themselves. However, more direct evidence supporting this hypothesis is needed.

Investigators have begun to examine expression of different NMDAR subunits following chronic EtOH exposure. Initial reports indicate that expression of NMDAR subunit mRNA increases following chronic EtOH exposure to neurons in culture as well as in brain tissue from rodents exposed to chronic EtOH treatment (Follesa and Ticku 1994; Bucci et al. 1993). These changes in receptor subunit expression may lead to alterations in receptor number or subunit constitution, both of which could have profound effects on glutamatergic synaptic transmission involving NMDA receptors.

Changes in NMDA receptor number or subunit composition following chronic EtOH exposure may also contribute to EtOH dependence and the neural changes underlying the EtOH withdrawal syndrome. Research to date has focused mainly on EtOH withdrawal, since this is easier to define operationally than dependence. It is reasonable to suspect the involvement of NMDA receptors in a number of the behavioral changes elicited by EtOH withdrawal in dependent animals. For example, withdrawal is anxiogenic, and severe convulsions can often be elicited in animals undergoing withdrawal (Adinoff et al. 1988; Lal et al. 1988; Hoffman et al. 1992). NMDA receptors are thought to play roles in both anxiogenesis and seizure development. Thus, it is possible that increased NMDA receptor activation during withdrawal contributes to both of these neural symptoms of withdrawal. The bulk of research to date has examined the role of NMDA receptors in EtOH withdrawal induced convulsions in mice and rats.

Treatment with NMDA receptor antagonists has been shown to reduce the severity of EtOH withdrawal induced convulsions in both mice (Grant et al. 1990) and rats (Morrisett et al. 1990; Morgan et al. 1992; Riaz and Faingold 1994). Activation of the receptor by administration of NMDA, on the other hand, appears to exacerbate withdrawal seizure severity and can render seizures intractable and lethal (Grant et al. 1990; Sanna et al. 1993). An interesting recent report indicates strong NMDA receptor activation in dentate gyrus and piriform cortex during withdrawal (Morgan et al. 1992). NMDA receptors have been implicated in processes underlying the production of audiogenic seizures during EtOH withdrawal in rats. Neuronal hyperexcitability in the inferior colliculus is one important neurophysiological event underlying audiogenic seizures (McCown et al. 1987; Riaz and Faingold 1994). Microinjection of NMDA receptor antagonists into the inferior colliculus can prevent audiogenic seizures while injection of NMDA will exacerbate seizures (Riaz and Faingold 1994). It is interesting to note that audiogenic EtOH withdrawal seizures in this brain region are also subject to the "kindling" phenomenon (McCown and Breese 1990). Kindling is a permanent enhancement of the ability of a particular brain region to exhibit epileptiform activity brought about by repeated elicitation of such activity in that brain region. In the case of the inferior colliculus and audiogenic withdrawal seizures, it is known that seizures induced by electrical stimulation are more likely to occur in animals which have undergone past withdrawal seizures, and that the reverse is also true. In addition, animals that have undergone past withdrawal seizures are more likely to exhibit audiogenic seizures after a given dose of EtOH than are naive animals (McCown and Breese 1990). NMDA receptor activation has been implicated in this kindling phenomenon as in kindling of handling-induced seizures during EtOH withdrawal (Becker and Hale 1993).

Studies of the genetic basis of EtOH withdrawal severity also support a role for NMDA receptors in the production of withdrawal-related neuronal hyperexcitability and convulsions. Differences in NMDA receptor number have been observed in animals selectively bred for differences in withdrawal seizure severity (the withdrawal seizure prone; WSP; and resistant; WSR; rats; Valverius et al. 1990). Effects of drugs with actions at the NMDA receptor also differ between withdrawal seizure prone and withdrawal seizure resistant rats (Crabbe et al. 1991). It is not yet clear whether NMDA receptor genes play any role in the genetic differences between these rat strains. A better understanding of the interstrain genetic differences that contribute to withdrawal seizure severity and identification and characterization of NMDA receptor subunit genes should aid in evaluating whether differences in NMDA receptors are a primary cause or a consequence of the genetic differences exhibited by these animals.

NMDA Receptors and Alcohol-Related Neuronal Damage

It is well known that chronic alcohol abuse can cause severe brain damage. There is evidence that alcohol-related brain damage involves both neuronal and glial cell damage (Charness 1993; Martin 1993). Ethanol itself does not appear to be a potent toxin for most neurons, with notable exceptions such as cerebellar granule cells (Scott et al. 1986; Pantazis et al. 1993; Heaton et al. 1994). If EtOH itself does not kill many types of neurons which are known to be susceptible to alcohol-related neurotoxicity in vivo, we must consider other factors associated with repeated ingestion of EtOH as possible causal agents or events. The following discussion focuses on excitotoxicity resulting from chronic alcohol abuse as there is now evidence linking NMDA receptor-induced excitotoxicity to neuronal cell death.

Excitotoxicity is the process whereby abnormally strong activation of neurons leads ultimately to neuronal death (see Shaw 1992; Choi 1988, 1994). The mechanisms involved in this form of neuropathology have been described extensively in the publications referenced above, and they are not disscussed in any detail here. It is clear that activation of glutamate receptors is one of the most powerful stimuli for initiating excitotoxicity in the brain. Studies of alcohol-related neurotoxicity have implicated NMDA receptor mediated excitotoxicity in alcohol-related brain damage involving nutritional deficits as well as toxicity which may be more directly related to the actions of alcohol (Lancaster 1992; Butterworth et al. 1993; Charness 1993; Lovinger 1993; Manzo et al. 1994; Tsai et al. 1995).

One undesirable outcome of prolonged EtOH exposure is thiamine deficiency which results from decreased thiamine intake and uptake as well as impaired utilization of this cofactor during prolonged periods of alcohol ingestion (see Butterworth et al. 1993; Charness 1993; Martin 1993; Manzo et al. 1994 for review). Indeed, it has long been known that thiamine deficiency is a major contributor to alcohol-induced Wernicke's encephalitis and Korsakoff's syndrome. However, the mechanisms linking thiamine deficiency to neurotoxicity are not well understood. Thiamine deficiency is known to lead to brain region selective neurotoxicity (Langlais et al. 1992; Butterworth 1993; Manzo et al. 1994). Recent studies have implicated excitotoxicity in selected brain regions in neuronal damage produced by thiamine deficiency (Langlais and Mair 1990; Langlais and Zhang 1993; Hazell et al. 1993). It was initially demonstrated that MK-801 could prevent thiamine deficiency induced loss of neurons in the thalamus and periaqueductal gray regions (Langlais and Mair 1990). This finding suggests that one of the events taking place during thiamine deficiency is enhanced activation of NMDA receptors. Increased glutamatergic transmission may underlie this increase in receptor activation. Indeed, experiments examining extracellular glutamate concentrations in different brain regions from thiamine-deficient rats have revealed increases in glutamate in vivo (Hazell et al. 1993; Langlais and Zhang 1993). Interestingly, these increases were seen prior to the development of neuronal loss but did appear to coincide with thiamine deficiency induced behavioral changes including loss of righting reflex (Hazell et al. 1993) and convulsions (Langlais and Zhang 1993). Increases in extracellular glutamate were observed in areas known to be susceptible to thiamine deficiency induced neuronal damage (medial thalamus) but not in regions where no evidence of neurotoxicity has been observed (dorsolateral thalamus, frontal parietal cortex). These findings suggest that increased release of glutamate either just before or during epileptiform activity may be one factor contributing to thiamine deficiency induced neuronal damage. Brain regional differences in glutamate release increases may underlie regional differences in susceptibility to neuronal toxicity. Increased glutamate release may not be the primary cause of regional differences in thiamine's neural actions. If the increase in extracellular glutamate develops only after seizure activity begins, this neurochemical change is likely secondary to another alteration brought about by thiamine deficiency. The identity of this more primary neuropathological change in the thiamine-deficient brain is an important target of continuing research.

The idea that excitotoxic mechanisms, possibly involving the NMDA receptor, might be involved in alcohol-induced brain damage independently of nutritional considerations has been put forward in recent publications (Lancaster 1992; Lovinger 1993; Hunt 1993). Readers are referred to these reviews for a more comprehensive discussion of this area. The present review concentrates on evidence from research performed since the publication of these articles. Briefly summarized, several investigators have postulated that excitotoxicity occurs when the brain is released from EtOH-induced inhibition and is then free to express hyperexcitability brought about by cellular and molecular changes which developed in adaptation to the depressant effects of EtOH. One of the suspected compensatory changes is an increase in NMDA receptor number, as discussed above. It is easy to imagine that the potential for excitotoxic damage would increase if the number of these receptors is increased since it is known that activation of NMDA receptors can lead to excitotoxicity. One prediction made from this postulate was that NMDA receptor mediated excitotoxicity would increase following chronic EtOH exposure. It has generally been observed that chronic exposure to EtOH increases the susceptibility of cultured cerebellar, cortical and hippocampal neurons to excitotoxicity produced by NMDA receptor activation (Iorio et al. 1993; Chandler et al. 1993; Smothers et al. 1995; Mirshahi et al. 1995). The increase in excitotoxicity appears to be selective for NMDA receptors since excitotoxicity produced by activation of other glutamate receptors is not altered following chronic EtOH exposure (Iorio et al. 1993; Smothers et al. 1995). It should be stressed that chronic exposure to EtOH at concentrations up to 100 m*M* is not toxic in and of itself. The increased toxicity is only observed when one activates the NMDA receptor. However, it is thought that increased receptor activation is brought about by the combination of glutamate release and increased NMDA receptor numbers following chronic EtOH exposure in vivo. The increased NMDA receptor mediated neurotoxicity following chronic EtOH exposure appears to be dependent on EtOH withdrawal. If EtOH is maintained in the environment during NMDA receptor activation following a 7 day exposure to EtOH, then one observes neuroprotection that is similar to that seen during acute EtOH exposure (Chandler et al. 1993). This observation is probably explained by the fact that EtOH inhibition of NMDA receptors is not lost following chronic alcohol exposure. Thus, NMDA receptor function and excitotoxicity would remain depressed during maintained chronic EtOH treatment. It is only after the inhibition by EtOH is removed and receptors are over-activated that the potential for enhanced excitotoxicity is fully relaized.

The potential role of increased NMDA receptor number has been stressed in the present discussion. However, we must not overlook other factors which could contribute to enhanced NMDA receptor mediated excitotoxicity following chronic EtOH exposure. Changes in NMDA receptor subunit composition might alter the potential of the receptor for initiating excitotoxicity. Different NMDA receptor subtypes do show differences in their time course of activation which might lead to differential entry of calcium during receptor activation (Monyer et al. 1994). There is good evidence that calcium entry is an important early event in receptor-mediated excitotoxicity (Choi 1988). Thus, differences in the amount of calcium entering following receptor activation might alter neuronal loss after chronic exposure. Changes in intracellular calcium dynamics such as loss of buffering might also be important. Alterations in calcium-dependent production of endogenous neurotoxins such as nitric oxide or hydroxyl or peroxyl radicals would also enhance excitotoxicity following NMDA receptor activation. This possibility is currently being investigated (Davda et al. 1993). However, it is not clear why NMDA receptor mediated excitotoxicity would be enhanced selectively by such changes. Increased release of glutamate might also contribute to enhanced toxicity, particularly in vivo. A recent preliminary study indicates that extracellular glutamate concentrations are increased many hours after EtOH withdrawal in rat hippocampus (Harms and Woodward 1995). Finally, I have previously discussed mechanisms by which changes in GABAergic inhibition could enhance NMDA receptor mediated signals following chronic EtOH exposure (Lovinger 1993). Such mechanisms would work to enhance NMDA receptor mediated excitotoxicity.

Potential for Pharmacotherapy Using Drugs Acting at the NMDA Receptor

From the foregoing review it would seem that agents with actions at the NMDA receptor could be useful in treating a variety of effects of EtOH. For example, NMDA receptor activation may reverse some aspects of acute intoxication or toxicity. NMDA receptor blockade might be useful in curbing the development of EtOH tolerance and might be used to prevent EtOH withdrawal convulsions and perhaps even alcohol-related brain damage. Studies in animal models have provided preliminary evidence of these potential therapeutic uses.

However, altering NMDA receptor function carries a considerable risk. Excessive NMDA receptor activation is convulsant in animals (see Grant et al. 1990a). NMDA and other receptor agonists are also known to be effective excitotoxins. Thus, one cannot administer NMDA receptor agonists or potentiating cofactors without the risk of convulsions and excitotoxicity.

The highly efficacious competitive and noncompetitive NMDA receptor antagonists also have undesirable side effects. Most notable in humans are the psychotomimetic effects of phencyclidine and related drugs. These unwanted effects include hallucinations, bizarre and unpredictable behaviors, and severe dysphoria (see Willetts et al. 1990; French et al. 1991; Meldrum 1992; Kornhuber and Weller 1993; Lipton 1993; Rogawski 1993; Patat et al. 1994 for discussion). In animal models NMDA receptor antagonists of many kinds elicit stereotypic behaviors which may indicate the presence of a psychotomimetic effect, cause motor impairment and have amnestic effects (Loscher and Honack 1991; De Sarro and De Sarro 1993; Murata and Kawasaki 1993). Thus, one cannot administer antagonists which block the effects of all forms of NMDA receptors without the risk of significant cognitive impairment. It is clear that considerable issues of safety are associated with the therapeutic use of NMDA receptor-acting agents.

Possible alternative therapies aimed at NMDA receptors are currently being explored with the goal of retaining pharmacotherapeutic efficacy with increased safety. One approach is to develop therapeutic agents which are selective for particular NMDA receptor subtypes. It is hoped that one can reduce the negative impact of NMDA receptor activation by eliminating the activation of a subpopulation of the receptors, but allow for enough receptor activation to subserve the necessary neural functions of the receptor. Since there is regional heterogeneity in the expression of NMDA receptor subunits, it is also possible that receptor subtype-specific agents might target particular brain regions. Ifenprodil is a subtype-selective NMDA receptor antagonist (Williams et al. 1993; Williams 1994; Lovinger 1995). This compound has been administered to humans and appears to be safe (see Caillard et al. 1993). Medicinal chemists have developed derivatives of this compound with high selectivity for NMDA receptors that may be clinically useful (Patat et al. 1994). The efficacy of these compounds for treatment of alcohol-related neural effects is not yet known. Another potentially useful approach is the development of agents with low efficacy at the receptor. One example is ADCI which produces only partial receptor antagonism even at relatively high concentrations (Grant et al. 1992). This agent has been shown to be efficacious in preventing EtOH withdrawal convulsions at concentrations that do not elicit evidence of motor impairment or stereotypic behaviors in animal models. Thus, this agent or a similar "partial antagonist" might have suitable efficacy for use in pharmacotherapy with higher safety than the more efficacious antagonists. Dextromethorphan, which has been used as a cough suppressant, also has antagonist actions at the NMDA receptor and does not appear to have psychotomimetic effects (Tortella et al. 1989). A final approach to the therapeutic use of NMDA receptor antagonists would be to use agents which target sites on the receptor that have allosteric effects on receptor function. These include drugs with actions on the glycine co-agonist site, the magnesium recognition site and sites at which polyamines have both positive and negative allosteric actions.

It is worth noting that some agents which have been used therapeutically have now been discovered to alter NMDA receptor function. Dextromethorphan and ifenprodil are examples of such drugs, and acamprosate may act on NMDA receptors as well. This latter drug has been used successfully to reduce alcohol intake in alcoholic humans with little evidence of unwanted behavioral side effects (Nalpas et al. 1990; Lhuintre et al. 1990; Gewiss et al. 1991; Moore and Libert 1991; Ades and Lejoyeux 1993). Recent evidence indicates that this compound can alter responses mediated by NMDA receptors in rat brain slices (Zeise et al. 1993). It will be interesting to examine the subtype specificity and efficacy of this compound.

Summary

Glutamatergic transmission involving NMDA receptors has now been implicated in a number of effects of acute and chronic EtOH exposure. Ethanol inhibits NMDA receptor function at intoxicating concentrations, and there is evidence that this inhibition contributes to acute EtOH intoxication. Chronic EtOH exposure leads to tolerance to and dependence on EtOH. Upregulation of NMDA receptor number or changes in receptor subunit composition may contribute to both of these adaptive processes. In addition, NMDA receptor activation appears to be involved in the development of EtOH tolerance. It is thought that NMDA receptor dependent synaptic plasticity is necessary for certain forms of tolerance. Supranormal activation of NMDA receptors is also implicated in alcohol-related brain damage. It has been hypothesized that NMDA receptor activation is increased during extended thiamine deficiency and after chronic EtOH exposure and withdrawal. The increased receptor activation is thought to lead to excitotoxicity and eventually to perceptible brain damage. Some support for the excitotoxicity hypothesis of alcohol-related brain damage has accumulated in recent studies utilizing animal and in vitro models. It is hoped that therapies targeting the NMDA receptor will be useful in preventing the undesirable effects of both acute and chronic EtOH exposure. However, significant side effects of drugs which act on the NMDA receptor must first be overcome.

References

Ades J, Lejoyeux M (1993) Clinical evaluation of acamprosate to reduce alcohol intake. Alcohol Alcohol 2: 275–278

Adinoff B, Bone GH, Linnoila M (1988) Acute ethanol poisoning and the ethanol withdrawal syndrome. Med Toxicol Adv Drug Exp 3(3): 172–196

Ahern KB, Lustig HS, Greenberg DA (1994) Enhancement of NMDA toxicity and calcium responses by chronic exposure of cultured neurons to ethanol. Neurosci Lett 165: 211–214

Alifimoff JK, Firestone LL, Miller KW (1989) Anaesthetic potencies of primary alkanols: implications for the molecular dimensions of the anaesthetic site. Br J Pharmacol 96(1): 9–16
Allan AM, Harris RA (1987) Involvement of neuronal chloride channels in ethanol intoxication, tolerance, and dependence. In: Galanter M (ed) Recent developments in alcoholism. Plenum, New York, pp 313–322
Anantharam V, Panchal RG, Wilson A, Kolchine VV, Treistman SN, Bayley H (1992) Combinatorial RNA splicing alters the surface charge on the NMDA receptor. FEBS Lett 305(1): 27–30
Andreasen M, Lambert JDC, Jensen MS (1989) Effects of new non-N-methyl-D-aspartate antagonists on synaptic transmission in the in vitro rat hippocampus. J Physiol (Lond) 414: 317–336
Balster RL, Grech DM, Bobelis DJ (1992) Drug discrimination analysis of ethanol as an N-methyl-D-aspartate receptor antagonist. Eur J Pharmacol 222: 39–42
Barnes JM, Henley JM (1992) Molecular characteristics of excitatory amino acid receptors. Prog Neurobiol 39(2): 113–133
Becker HC, Hale RL (1993) Repeated episodes of ethanol withdrawal potentiate the severity of subsequent withdrawal seizures: an animal model of alcohol withdrawal "kindling". Alcohol Clin Exp Res 17(1): 94–98
Blitzer RD, Gil O, Landau EM (1990) Long-term potentiation in rat hippocampus is inhibited by low concentrations of ethanol. Brain Res 537: 203–208
Boren JL, Consroe P (1981) Phencyclidine (PCP) and ethanol: potentiation of lethality and sleep time with combined administration in rats. Neurobehav Toxicol Teratol 3: 11–14
Brunet BL, Reiffenstein RJ, Williams T, Wong L (1986) Toxicity of phencyclidine and ethanol in combination. Alcohol Drug Res 6: 341–349
Bucci DJ, Keir WJ, Morrow AL (1993) Effect of chronic ethanol administration on NMDAR1-receptor subunit mRNA levels. Soc Neurosci Abstr 19: 378
Buck KJ, Harris RA (1991) Neuroadaptive responses to chronic ethanol. Alcohol Clin Exp Res 15: 460–470
Buller AL, Morrisett RA, Seeburg PH, Monaghan DT (1993) Interaction of ethanol (EtOH) with recombinant heteromeric NMDA receptors expressed in Xenopus oocytes. Alcohol Clin Exp Res 17(2): 475
Butelman ER, Baron SP, Woods JH (1993) Ethanol effects in pigeons trained to discriminate MK-801, PCP or CGS-19755. Behav Parmacol 4: 57–60
Butterworth RF (1993) Pathophysiology of cerebellar dysfunction in the Wernicke-Korsakoff syndrome. Can J Neurol Sci 20(3): S123–126
Butterworth RF, Kril JJ, Harper CG (1993) Thiamine-dependent enzyme changes in the brains of alcoholics: relationship to the Wernicke-Korsakoff syndrome. Alcohol Clin Exp Res 17(5): 1084–1088
Caillard P, Mouren X, Bailliart O, Cloarec M (1993) Evaluation of ifenprodil efficacy on exercise-induced tissue ischemia in stage II arteriopathy by measurement of transcutaneous oxygen tension during a standard treadmill test: double-blind study of injectable ifenprodil versus placebo. Angiology 44(7): 552–560
Carmignoto G, Vicini S (1992) Activity-dependent decrease in NMDA receptor responses during development of the visual cortex. Science 258(5084): 1007–1011
Chait LD, Wenger GR, McMillan DE (1981) Effects of phencyclidine and ketamine on punished and unpunished responding by pigeons. Pharmacol Biochem Behav 15: 145–148
Chandler LJ, Newsom H, Sumners C, Crews F (1993) Chronic ethanol exposure potentiates NMDA excitotoxicity in cerebral cortical neurons. J Neurochem 60(4): 1578–1581
Chandler LJ, Guzman NJ, Sumners C, Crews FT (1994) Magnesium and zinc potentiate ethanol inhibition of N-methyl-D-aspartate-stimulated nitric oxide synthase in cortical neurons. J Pharmacol Exp Ther 271(1): 67–75
Charness ME (1993) Brain lesions in alcoholics. Alcohol Clin Exp Res 17(1): 2–11
Choi DW (1988) Glutamate neurotoxicity and diseases of the nervous system. Neuron 1: 623–634
Choi DW (1994) Glutamate receptors and the induction of excitotoxic neuronal death. Prog Brain Res 100: 47–51
Clineschmidt BV, Martin GE, Bunting PR (1982) Anticonvulsant activity of (+)-5-methyl-10, 11-dihydro-5H-dibenzo[a,d] cyclohepten-5,10-imine (MK-801), a substance with potent anticonvulsant, central sympathomimetic, and apparent anxiolytic properties. Drug Dev Res 2: 123–134
Collingridge GL, Bliss TVP (1987) NMDA receptors: Their role in long-term potentiation. Trends Neurosci 10: 288–293
Crabbe JC, Merrill CD, Belknap JK (1991) Effects of convulsants on handling-induced convulsions in mice selected for ethanol withdrawal severity. Brain Res 550(1): 1–6

Criado JR, Steffensen SC, Henriksen SJ (1994) Ethanol acts via the ventral tegmental area to influence hippocampal physiology. Synapse 17(2): 84–91
Danysz W, Dyr W, Jankowska E, Glazewski S, Kostowski W (1992) The involvement of NMDA receptors in acute and chronic effects of ethanol. Alcohol Clin Exp Res 16(3): 499–504
Davda RK, Chandler LJ, Crews FT, Guzman NJ (1993) Ethanol enhances the endothelial nitric oxide synthase response to agonists. Hypertension 21(2): 939–943
De Sarro GB, De Sarro A (1993) Anticonvulsant properties of non-competitive antagonists of the N-methyl-D-aspartate receptor in genetically epilepsy-prone rats: comparison with CPPene. Neuropharmacology 32(1): 51–58
Devenport LD, Merriman VJ (1983) Ethanol and behavioral variability in the radial-arm maze. Psychopharmacology 79(1): 21–24
Dietrich RA (1987) Interaction of ethanol with other drugs. In: Galanter M (ed) Recent developments in alcoholism, vol 5. Plenum, New York, pp 283–301
Dietrich RA, Dunwiddie TV, Harris RA, Erwin VG (1989) Mechanism of action of ethanol: initial central nervous system actions. Pharmacol Rev 41: 489–537
Dildy JE, Leslie SW (1989) Ethanol inhibits NMDA-induced increases in intracellular Ca^{2+} in dissociated brain cells. Brain Res 499: 383–387
Dildy-Mayfield JE, Harris RA (1992a) Acute and chronic ethanol alters the function of hippocampal kainate receptors expressed in *Xenopus* oocytes. J Neurochem 58: 1569–1572
Dildy-Mayfield JE, Harris RA (1992b) Comparison of ethanol sensitivity of rat brain kainate, DL-a-amino-3-hydroxy-5-methyl-4-isoxalone proprionic acid and N-methyl-D-aspartate receptors expressed in *Xenopus* oocytes. J Pharmacol Exp Ther 262: 487–494
Dildy-Mayfield JE, Leslie SW (1991) Mechanism of inhibition of N-methyl-D-aspartate-stimulated increases in free intracellular Ca^{2+} concentration by ethanol. J Neurochem 56: 1536–1543
Dolin S, Little H, Hudspith M et al (1987) Increased dihydropyridine-sensitive calcium channels in rat brain may underlie ethanol physical dependence. Neuropharmacology 26: 275–279
Dow KE, Riopelle RJ (1990) Ethanol inhibits NMDA-stimulated neurite growth by sensory neurons. Neuroreport 1(2): 111–114
Durand GM, Gregor P, Zheng X, Bennett MVL, Uhl GR, Zukin RS (1992) Cloning of an apparent splice variant of the rat N-methyl-D-aspartate receptor NMDAR1 with altered sensitivity to polyamines and activators of protein kinase C. Proc Natl Acad Sci USA 89: 9359–9363
Eberwine J, Yeh H, Miyashiro K, Cao Y, Nair S, Finnel R, Zattel M, Coleman P (1992) Analysis of gene expression in single live neurons. Proc Natl Acad Sci USA 89: 3010–3014
Fidecka S, Langwinski R (1989) Interaction between ketamine and EtOH in rats and mice, Pol J Pharmacol Pharm 41: 23–32
Fink K, Gothert M (1990) Inhibition of N-methyl-D-aspartate-induced noradrenaline release by alcohols is related to their hydrophobicity. Eur J Pharm 191(2): 225–229
Follesa P and Ticku MK (1994) Chronic ethanol administration differentially regulates NMDA receptor R1 and R2 subunit mRNAs in rat brain. Soc Neurosci Abstr 20: 494
Franks NP, Lieb WR (1985) Mapping of general anaesthetic target sites provides a molecular basis for cutoff effects. Nature 316(6026): 349–351
French ED, Ferkany J, Abreu M, Levenson S (1991) Effects of competitive N-methyl-D-aspartate antagonists on midbrain dopamine neurons: an electrophysiological and behavioral comparison to phencyclidine. Neuropharmacology 30(10): 1039–1046
Gewiss M, Heidbreder C, Opsomer L, Durbin P, De Witte P (1991) Acamprosate and diazepam differentially modulate alcohol-induced behavioural and cortical alteriations in rats following chronic inhalation of ethanol vapour. Alcohol Alcohol 26(2): 129–137
Gibson, WE (1985) Effects of alcohol on radial maze performance in rat. Physiol Behav 35: 1003–1005
Givens B (1995) Low doses of ethanol impair spatial working memory and reduce hippocampal theta activity. Alcohol Clin Exp Res 19(3): 763–767
Gonzales RA, Westbrook SL, Bridges LT (1991) Alcohol-induced inhibition of N-methyl-D-aspartate-evoked release of [3H] norepinephrine from brain is related to lipophilicity. Neuropharmacology 30(5): 441–446
Gordon A, Sapru MK, Krauss SW, Diamond I (1993) Nucleoside transport and ethanol-induced heterologous desensitization. In: Alling C, Diamond I, Leslie SW, Sun GY, Wood WG (eds) Alcohol, cell membranes, and signal transduction in brain. Plenum, New York, pp 195–204

Göthert M, Fink K (1989) Inhibition of N-methyl-D-aspartate (NMDA)- and l-glutamate-induced noradrenaline and acetylcholine release in the rat brain by EtOH. Naunyn Schmiedebergs Arch Pharmacol 340(5): 516–521
Grant KA, Colombo G (1993a) Discriminative stimulus effects of ethanol: Effects of training dose on the substitution of N-methyl-D-aspartate antagonists. J Pharmacology Exp Ther 264: 1241–1247
Grant KA, Colombo G (1993b) Pharmacological analysis of the mixed discriminative stimulus effects of ethanol. Alcohol Alcohol [Suppl] 2: 445–449
Grant KA, Hoffman PL, Tabakoff B (1990a) Neurobiological and behavioral approaches to tolerance and dependence. In: Edwards G, Lader M (eds) The nature of dependence. Oxford University Press, Oxford, pp 135–169
Grant KA, Knisely JS, Tabakoff B, Barrett JE, Balster, RL (1991) Ethanol-like discriminative stimulus effects of noncompetitive N-methyl-D-aspartate antagonists. Behav Pharmacol 2: 87–95
Grant KA, Snell LD, Rogawski MA, Thurkauf A, Tabakoff B (1992) Comparison of the effects of the uncompetitive N-methyl-D-aspartate antagonist (+)-5-aminocarbonyl-10,11-dihydro-5H-dibenzo [a,d] cyclohepten-5,10-imine (ADCI) with its structural analogs dizocilpine (MK-801) and carbamazepine on ethanol withdrawal seizures. J Pharmacol Exp Ther 260(3): 1017–1022
Grant KA, Valverius P, Hudspith M, Tabakoff B (1990b) Ethanol withdrawal seizures and the NMDA receptor complex. Eur J Pharm 176(3): 289–296
Greenamyre JT, Porter RH (1994) Anatomy and physiology of glutamate in the CNS. Neurology 44(11): S7-13
Greenberg DA, Carpenter CL, Messing RO (1987) Ethanol-induced component of 45Ca2+ uptake in PC12 cells is sensitive to Ca2+ channel modulating drugs. Brain Res 410: 143–146
Grover CA, Frye GD, Griffith WH (1994) Acute tolerance to ethanol inhibition of NMDA-mediated EPSPs in the CA1 region of the rat hippocampus. Brain Res 642(1-2): 70–76
Guimaraes FS, Carobrez AP, DeAguiar JC, Graeff FG (1991) Anxiolytic effect in the elevated plus-maze of the NMDA receptor antagonist AP7 microinjected into the dorsal periaqueductal grey. Psychopharmacology 103: 91–94
Gulya K, Grant KA, Valverius P, Hoffman PL, Tabakoff B (1991) Brain regional specificity and time course of changes in the NMDA receptor-ionophore complex during ethanol withdrawal. Brain Res 547: 129–134
Harms JF, Woodward JJ (1995) Efflux of excitatory amino acids in the rat hippocampus during withdrawal from chronic ethanol as measured by in vivo microdialysis. Alcohol Clin Exp Res 19(2): 5A
Hazell AS, Butterworth RF, Hakim AM (1993) Cerebral vulnerability is associated with selective increase in extracellular glutamate concentration in experimental thiamine deficiency. J Neurochem 61(3): 1155–1158
Heaton MB, Paiva M, Swanson DJ, Walker DW (1994) Ethanol neurotoxicity in vitro: effects of GM1 ganglioside and protein synthesis inhibition. Brain Res 654: 336–342
Hestrin S (1992) Developmental regulation of NMDA receptor-mediated synaptic currents at a central synapse. Nature 357(6380): 686–689
Hoffman P, Grant KA, Snell LD, Reinlib L, Iorio K, Tabakoff B (1992) NMDA receptors: role in ethanol withdrawal seizures. Ann NY Acad Sci 654: 52–60
Hoffman PL, Rabe CS, Moses F, Tabakoff B (1989a) N-methyl-D-aspartate receptors and ethanol: inhibition of calcium flux and cyclic GMP production. J Neurochem 52: 1937–1940
Hoffman PL, Moses F, Tabakoff B (1989b) Selective inhibition by ethanol of glutamate-stimulated cyclic GMP production in primary cultures of cerebellar granule cells. Neuropharmacology 28: 1239–1243
Hollmann M, Heinemann S (1994) Cloned glutamate receptors. Annu Rev Neurosci 17: 31–108
Huettner JE, Bean BP (1988) Block of N-methyl-D-aspartate-activated current by the anticonvulsant MK-801: selective binding to open channels. Proc Natl Acad Sci USA 85(4): 1307–1311
Hunt WA (1993) Are binge drinkers more at risk of developing brain damage? Alcohol 10(6): 559–561
Iorio KR, Reinlib L, Tabakoff B, Hoffman PL (1992) Chronic exposure of cerebellar granule cells to ethanol results in increased N-methyl-D-aspartate receptor function. Mol Pharmacol 41: 1142–1148
Iorio KR, Tabakoff B, Hoffman PL (1993) Glutamate-induced neurotoxicity is increased in cerebellar granule cells exposed chronically to ethanol. Eur J Pharmacol 248: 209–212

Ishii T, Moriyoshi H, Sugihara H, Sakurada K, Kadotani H, Yokoi M, Akazawa C, Shigemoto R, Mizuno N, Masu M, Nakanishi S (1993) Molecular characterization of the family of the N-methyl-D-aspartate receptor subunits. J Biol Chem 268: 2836–2843
Jahr CE, Stevens CF (1993) Calcium permeability of the N-methyl-D-aspartate receptor channel in hippocampal neurons in culture. Proc Natl Acad Sci USA 90(24): 11573–11577
Jonas P, Spruston N (1994) Mechanisms shaping glutamate-mediated excitatory postsynaptic currents in the CNS. Curr Opin Neurobiol 4(3): 366–372
Jones RW, Leslie SW (1993) Inhibition by ethanol of the D, L-(tetrazol-5-YL) glycine stimulation of the N-methyl-D-aspartate receptor in a rat brain dissociated cell preparation. Alcohol Clin Exp Res 17(2): 474
Kalant H (1993) Problems in the search for mechanisms of tolerance. Alcohol Alcohol 2: 1–8
Keinanen K, Wisden W, Sommer B, Werner P, Herb A, Verdoorn TA, Sakmann B, Seeburg PH (1990) A family of AMPA-selective glutamate receptors. Science 249(4968): 556–560
Khanna JM, Shah G, Weiner J, Wu PH, Kalant H (1993) Effect of NMDA receptor antagonists on rapid tolerance to ethanol. Eur J Pharmacol 230(1): 23–31
Khanna JM, Morato GS, Chau A, Shah G, Kalant H (1994) Effect of NMDA antagonists on rapid and chronic tolerance to ethanol: importance of intoxicated practice. Pharmacol Biochem Behav 48(3): 755–763
Koltchine V, Anantharam V, Wilson A, Bayley H, Treistman SN (1993) Homomeric assemblies of NMDAR1 splice variants are sensitive to ethanol. Neurosci Lett 152: 13–16
Komuro H, Rakic P (1993) Modulation of neuronal migration by NMDA receptors. Science 260(5104): 95–97
Koob GF (1992) Neural mechanisms of drug reinforcement. Ann NY Sci 654: 171–191
Koob GF, Bloom FE (1988) Cellular and molecular mechanisms of drug dependence. Science 242(4879): 715–723
Kornhuber J, Weller M (1993) Amantadine and the glutamate hypothesis of schizophrenia. Experiences in the treatment of neuroleptic malignant syndrome. J Neural Trans 92(1): 57–65
Kuner T, Schoepfer R, Korpi ER (1993) Ethanol inhibits glutamate-induced currents in heteromeric NMDA receptor subtypes. Neuroreport 5(3): 237–300
Kutsuwada T, Kashiwabuchi N, Morei J, Sakimura K, Kushiya E, Araki K, Meguro H, Masaki J, Kumanishi T, Arakawa M, Mishina M (1992) Molecular diversity of the NMDA receptor channel. Nature 358: 36–41
Lal H, Harris CM, Springfield AC, Bhadra S, Emmett-Oglesby MW (1988) Characterization of a pentylenetetrazol-like interoceptive stimulus produced by ethanol withdrawal. Pharmacol Exp Ther 247: 508–518
Lancaster FE (1992) Alcohol, nitric oxide, and neurotoxicity: is there a connection? Alcohol Clin Exp Res 16(3): 539–541
Langlais PJ, Mair RG (1990) Protective effects of the glutamate antagonist MK-801 on pyrithiamine-induced lesions and amino acid changes in rat brain. J Neurosci 10(5): 1664–1674
Langlais PJ, Zhang SX (1993) Extracellular glutamate is increased in thalamus during thiamine deficiency-induced lesions and is blocked by MK-801. J Neurochem 61(6): 2175–2182
Langlais PJ, Mandel RJ, Mair RG (1992) Diencephalic lesions, learning impairments, and intact retrograde memory following acute thiamine deficiency in the rat. Behav Brain Res 48(2): 177–185
Lhuintre JP, Moore N, Tran G, Steru L, Langrenon S, Daoust M, Parot P, Ladure P, Libert C, Boismare F, Hillemand B (1990) Acamprosate appears to decrease alcohol intake in weaned alcoholics. Alcohol Alcohol 25(6): 613–622
Liebman JM, Bennett DA (1988) Anxiolytic actions of competitive N-methyl-D-aspartate receptor antagonists: a comparison with benzodiazepine modulators and dissociative anesthetics. In: Cavalheiro EH, Lehmann J, Turski L (eds) Frontiers in excitatory amino acid research. Liss, New York, pp 301–308
Lima-Landman MTR, Albuquerque EX (1989) Ethanol potentiates and blocks NMDA-activated single-channel currents in rat hippocampal pyramidal cells. FEBS Lett 247: 61–67
Linden DJ (1994) Long-term synaptic depression in the mammalian brain. Neuron 12(3): 457–472
Lipton SA (1993) Prospects for clinically tolerated NMDA antagonists: open-channel blockers and alternative redox states of nitric oxide. Trends Neurosci 16(12): 527–532
Lister RG, Eckardt M, Weinggartner H (1987) Ethanol intoxication and memory. Recent developments and new directions, In: Galanter M (ed) Recent developments in alcoholism, vol 5. Plenum, New York, pp 111–125

Lodge D, Aram JA, Church J, Davies SN, Martin D, O'Shaughnessy CT, Zeman S (1987) Excitatory amino acids and phencyclidine-like drugs. In: Hicks TP, Lodge D, McLennan H (eds) Excitatory amino acid transmission. Liss, New York, pp 83–90
Loscher W, Honack D (1991) Anticonvulsant and behavioral effects of two novel competitive N-methyl-D-aspartic acid receptor antagonists, CGP 37849 and CGP 39551, in the kindling model of epilepsy. Comparison with MK-801 and carbamazepine. J Pharmacol Exp Ther 256(2):432–440
Lovinger DM (1993) Excitotoxicity and alcohol-related brain damage. Alcohol Clin Exp Res 17: 19–27
Lovinger DM (1995) Developmental decrease in ethanol inhibition of N-methyl-D-aspartate receptors in rat neocortical neurons: relation to the actions of ifenprodil. J Pharmacol Exp Ther 274: 164–172
Lovinger DM, Grant KA (1995) Alcohol neurotoxicity: effects and mechanisms. In: Chang LW, Dyer RS (eds) Handbook of neurotoxicology. Dekker, New York, pp 769–800
Lovinger DM, Peoples RW (1993) Actions of alcohols and other sedative/hypnotic compounds on cation channels associated with glutamater and 5-HT3 receptors. In: Alling C, Diamond I, Leslie SW, Sun GY, Wood WG (eds) Alcohol, cell membranes, and signal transduction in brain. Plenum, New York, pp 157–168
Lovinger DM, White G, Weight FF (1989) Ethanol inhibits NMDA-activated ion current in hippocampal neurons. Science 243: 1721–1724
Lovinger DM, White G, Weight FF (1990) NMDA receptor-mediated synaptic excitation selectively inhibited by ethanol in hippocampal slice from adult rat. J Neurosci 10(4): 1372–1379
MacDermott AB, Dale N (1987) Receptors, ion channels and synaptic potentials underlying the integrative actions of excitatory amino acids. Trends Neurosci 10: 280–284
MacDermott AB, Mayer ML, Westbrook GL, Smith SJ, Barker JL (1986) NMDA-receptor activation increases cytoplasmic calcium concentration in cultured spinal cord neurones. Nature 321(6069): 519–522
Manzo L, Locatelli C, Candura SM, Costa LG (1994) Nutrition and alcohol neurotoxicity. Neurotoxicology 15(3): 555–65
Martin D, Morrisett RA, Bian X-P, Wilson W, Swartzwelder HS (1991) Ethanol inhibition of NMDA mediated depolarizations is increased in the presence of Mg^{2+}. Brain Res 546: 227–234
Masood K, Wu C, Brauneis U, Weight FF (1994) Differential ethanol sensitivity of recombinant N-methyl-D-aspartate receptor subunits. Mol Pharmacol 45: 324–329
Matthews DB, Simson PE, Best PJ (1994) Ethanol disrupts activity of hippocampal "place cells" in awake behaving rats. Alcohol Clin Exp Res 18(2): 520
Matthews DB, Simson PE, Best PJ (1995) Acute ethanol impairs spatial memory but not stimulus/response memory in the rat. Alcohol Clin Exp Res 19: 902–909
Mayer ML, Westbrook GL (1987a) The physiology of excitatory amino acids in the vertebrate central nervous system. Prog Neurobiol 28(3): 197–276
Mayer ML, Westbrook GL (1987b) Permeation and block of N-methyl-D-aspartic acid receptor channels by divalent cations in mouse cultured central neurones. J Physiol (Lond) 394: 501–527
Mayer ML, MacDermott AB, Westbrook GL, Smith SJ, Barker JL (1987) Agonist- and voltagegated calcium entry in cultured mouse spinal cord neurons under voltage clamp measured using arsenazo III. J Neurosci 7(10): 3230–3244
Mayer ML, Vyklicky L, Sernagor E (1989) A Physiologists view on the N-methyl-D-aspartate receptor: an allosteric ion channel with multiple regulatory sites. Drug Dev Res 17: 263–280
McCown TJ, Breese GR (1990) Multiple withdrawals from chronic ethanol "kindles" inferior collicular seizure activity: evidence for kindling of seizures associated with alcoholism. Alcohol Clin Exp Res 14(3): 394–399
McCown TJ, Givens BS, Breese GR (1987) Amino acid influences on seizures elicited within the inferior colliculus. J Pharmacol Exp Ther 243(2): 603–608
Meguro H, Mori H, Araki K, Kushiya E, Kutsuwada T, Yamazki M, Kumanishi T, Arakawa M, Sakimura K, Mishina M (1992) Functional characterization of a heteromeric NMDA receptor channel expressed from cloned cDNAs. Nature 357: 70–74
Meldrum BS (1992) Excitatory amino acids in epilepsy and potential novel therapies. Epilepsy Res 12(2): 189–196
Mhatre MC, Ticku MK (1993) Alcohol: effects on GABAA receptor function and gene expression. In: Alling C, Diamond I, Leslie SW, Sun GY, Wood WG (eds) Alcohol, cell membranes, and signal trandsduction in brain. Plenum, New York, pp 175–184

Michaelis EK, Michaelis ML, Freed WJ, Foye J (1993) Glutamate receptor changes in brain synaptic membranes during chronic alcohol intake. Alcohol Alcohol 2: 377–381
Miller KW (1993) Multiple actions of ethanol on acetylcholine receptors. In: Alling C, Diamond I, Leslie SW, Sun GY, Wood WG (eds) Alcohol, cell membranes, and signal transduction in brain. Plenum, New York, pp 83–96
Mirshahi T, Woodward JJ (1995) Ethanol sensitivity of heteromeric NMDA receptors: effects of subunit assembly, glycine and NMDAR1 Mg^{2+} insensitive mutants. Neuropharmacology 34: 347–355
Mirshahi T, Blevins T, Woodward JJ (1995) Altered sensitivity of NMDA receptors to agonists and antagonists following chronic ethanol exposure. Alcohol Clin Exp Res 19(2): 5A
Montpied P, Morrow AL, Karanian JW et al. (1991) Prolonged ethanol inhalation decreases gamma-aminobutyric acid A receptor alpha subunit mRNA in the rat cerebral cortex. Mol Pharmacol 39: 158–163
Monyer H, Sprengel R, Schoepfer R, Herb A, Higuchi M, Lomeli H, Burnashev N, Sakmann B, Seeburg PH (1992) Heteromeric NMDA receptors: molecular and functional distinction of subtypes. Science 256: 1217–1221
Monyer H, Burnashev N, Laurie DJ, Sakmann B, Seeburg P (1994) Developmental and regional expression in the rat brain and functional properties of four NMDA receptors. Neuron 12: 529–540
Moore N, Libert C (1991) Acamprosate, citalopram, and alcoholism. Lancet 337(8751): 1228
Morgan PF, Nadi NS, Karanian J, Linnoila M (1992) Mapping rat brain structures activated during ethanol withdrawal-Role of glutamate and NMDA receptors. Eur J Pharmacol 225: 217–223
Moriyoshi K, Masu M, Kshii T, Shigemoto R, Mizuno N, Nakaniski S (1991) Molecular cloning and characterization of the rat NMDA receptor. Nature 354: 31–37
Morris RGM, Anderson E, Lynch GS, Baudry M (1986) Selective impairment of learning and blockade of long-term potentiation by an N-methyl-D-aspartate receptor antagonist, AP5. Nature 319: 774–776
Morrisett RA, Rezvani AH, Overstreet D, Janowsky DS, Wilson WA, Swartzwelder HS (1990) MK-801 potently inhibits alcohol withdrawal seizures in rats. Eur J Pharmacol 176: 103–105
Morrisett RA, Swartzwelder HS (1993) Attenuation of hippocampal long-term potentiation by ethanol: a patch-clamp analysis of glutamatergic and GABAergic mechanisms. J Neurosci 13(5): 2264–72
Morrisett RA, Martin D, Oetting TA, Lewis DV, Wilson WA, Swartzwelder HS (1991) Ethanol and magnesium ions inhibit N-methyl-D-aspartate-mediated synaptic potentials in an interactive manner. Neuropharmacology 30: 1173–1178
Morrow AL, Suzdak PD, Karanian JW, Paul SM (1988) Chronic ethanol administration alters gamma-aminobutyric acid, pentobarbital and ethanol-mediated 36Cl-uptake in cerebral cortical synaptoneurosomes. J Pharmacol Exp Ther 246: 158–164
Mulkeen D, Anwyl R, Rowan MJ (1987) Enhancement of long-term potentiation by the calcium channel agonist Bayer K8644 in CA1 of the rat hippocampus in vitro. Neurosci Lett 80: 351–355
Murata S, Kawasaki K (1993) Common and uncommon behavioural effects of antagonists for different modulatory sites in the NMDA receptor/channel complex. Eur J Pharmacol 239(1-3): 9–15
Nakanishi S (1994) The molecular diversity of glutamate receptors. Prog Clin Biol Res 390: 85–98
Nalpas B, Dabadie H, Parot P, Paccalin J (1990) L'acamprosate. De la pharmacologie à la clinique. Encephale 16(3): 175–179
Pantazis NJ, Dohrman DP, Goodlett CR, Cook RT, West JR (1993) Vulnerability of cerebellar granule cells to alcohol-induced cell death diminishes with time in culture. Alcohol Clin Exp Res 17: 1014–1021
Patat A, Molinier P, Hergueta T, Brohier S, Zieleniuk I, Danjou P, Warot D, Puech A (1994) Lack of amnestic, psychotomimetic or impairing effect on psychomotor performance of eliprodil, a new NMDA antagonist. Int Clin Psychopharmacol 9(3): 155–162
Peoples RW, Weight FF (1992) Ethanol inhibition of N-methyl-D-aspartate-activated ion current in rat hippocampal neurons is not competitive with glycine. Brain Res 571: 342–344
Peoples RW, Weight FF (1995) Cutoff in potency implicates alcohol inhibition of N-methyl-D-aspartate receptors in alcohol intoxication. Proc Natl Acad Sci USA 92(7): 2825–2829
Rabe CS, Tabakoff B (1990) Glycine site-directed agonists reverse the action of ethanol at the N-methyl-D-aspartame receptor. Mol Pharmacol 38: 753–757

Raditsch M, Ruppersberg JP, Kuner T, Gunther W, Schoepfer R, Seeburg PH, Jahn W, Witzemann V (1993) Subunit-specific block of cloned NMDA receptors by argiotoxin 636. FEBS Lett 324(1): 63–66
Raines DE, Korten SE, Hill AG, Miller KW (1993) Anesthetic cutoff in cycloalkanemethanols. A test of current theories. Anesthesiology 78(5): 918–927
Riaz A, Faingold CL (1994) Seizures during ethanol withdrawal are blocked by focal microinjection of excitant amino acid antagonists into the inferior colliculus and pontine reticular formation. Alcohol Clin Exp Res 18(6): 1456–1462
Rogawski MA (1993) Therapeutic potential of excitatory amino acid antagonists: channel blockers and 2, 3-benzodiazepines. Trends Pharmacol Sci 14(9): 325–331
Rogers J, Siggins GR, Schulman JA, Bloom FE (1979) Physiological correlates of ethanol intoxication, tolerance, and dependence in rat cerebellar Purkinje cells. Brain Res 196: 183–198
Samson HH, Harris RA (1992) Neurobiology of alcohol abuse. Trends Pharmacol Sci 13: 206–211
Sanger DJ (1993) Substitution by NMDA antagonists and other drugs in rats trained to discriminate ethanol. Behav Pharmacol 4: 523–528
Sanna E, Harris RA (1993) Neuronal ion channels. In: Galanter M (ed) Recent developments in alcoholism, vol 11: Ten years of progress. Plenum, New York, pp 169–186
Sanna E, Serra M, Cossu A, Colombo G, Follesa P, Cuccheddu T, Concas A, Biggio G. (1983) Chronic ethanol intoxication induces differential effects on GABAA and NMDA receptor function in the rat brain. Alcohol Clin Exp Res 17(1): 115–23
Schoepfer R, Monyer H, Sommer B, Wisden W, Sprengel R, Kuner T, Lomeli H, Herb A, Kohler M, Burnashev N et al (994) Molecular biology of glutamate receptors. Prog Neurobiol 42(2): 353–357
Schuckit MA (1995) Drug and alcohol abuse: a clinical guide to diagnosis and treatment. Plenum, New York
Scott B, Petit TL, Lew RJ (1986) Differential survival of fetal and adult neurons and nonneuronal cells exposed chronically to ethanol in cell culture. Neurotoxicology 7: 81–90
Seeburg PH (1993) The molecular biology of mammalian glutamate receptor channels. Trends Pharmacol Sci 14: 297–302
Shaw PJ (1992) Excitatory amino acid neurotransmission, excitotoxicity and excitotoxins. Curr Opin Neurol Neurosurg 5(3): 383–390
Shefner SA (1990) Electrophysiological effects of ethanol on brain neurons. In: Watson RR (ed) Biochemistry and physiology of substance abuse, vol II. CRC Press, Boca Raton, pp 25–52
Sheng M, Cummings J, Roldan LA, Jan YN, Jan LY (1994) Changing subunit composition of heteromeric NMDA receptors during development of rat cortex. Nature 368(6467): 144–147
Siggins GR, Pittman QJ, French ED (1987) Effects of ethanol on CA1 and CA3 pyramidal cells in the hippocampal slice preparation: an intracellular study. Brain Res 414: 22–34
Simsom PE, Criswell HE, Breese GR (1993) Inhibition of NMDA-evoked electrophysiological activity by ethanol in selected brain regions: evidence for ethanol-sensitive and ethanol-insensitive NMDA-evoked responses. Brain Res 607: 9–16
Sinclair JG, Lo GF (1986) Ethanol blocks tetanic and calcium-induced long-term potentiation in the hippocampal slice. Gen Pharmacol 17(2): 231–233
Skattebol A, Rabin RA (1987) Effects of ethanol on 45Ca2+ uptake in synaptosomes and in PC12 cells. Biochem Parmacol 36(13): 2227–2229
Smothers C, Mrotek J, Lovinger DM (1995) Chronic exposure to ethanol produces an enhancement of NMDA toxicity in cultured hippocampal neurons. Alcohol Clin Exp Res 19(2): 5A
Steffensen SC, Yeckel MF, Miller DR, Henriksen SJ (1993) Ethanol-induced suppression of hippocampal long-term potentiation is blocked by lesions of the septohippocampal nucleus. Alcohol Clin Exp Res 17(3): 655–659
Sugihara H, Moriyoshi K, Ishii T, Masu M, Nakanishi S (1992) Structure and properties of seven isoforms of the NMDA receptor generated by alternative splicing. Biochem Biophys Res Commun 185: 826–832
Sun G.Y, Zhang J, Lin T (1993) Effects of acute and chronic ethanol administration on the poly-phosphoinositide signaling activity in brain. In: Alling C, Diamond I, Leslie SW, Sun GY, Wood WG (ed) Alcohol, cell membranes, and signal transduction in brain. Plenum, New York, pp 205–218
Szabo G, Tabakoff B, Hoffman PL (1994) The NMDA receptor antagonist, dizocilpine, differentially affects environment-dependent and environment-independent ethanol tolerance. Psychopharmacology 113: 511–517
Tabakoff B, Hoffman PL (1988) Tolerance and etiology of alcoholism; hypothesis and mechanisms. Alcohol Clin Exp Res 12: 184–186

Tabakoff B, Hoffman PL (1995) Effect of alcohol on neurotransmitters and their receptors and enzymes. In: Begleiter H, Kissin B (ed) Alcohol and alcoholism, vol 2. Oxford University Press, New York
Tortella FC, Pellicano M, Bowery NG (1989) Dextromethorphan and neuromodulation: old drug coughs up new activities. Trends Pharmacol Sci 10(12): 501–507
Tremwel MF, Anderson KJ, Hunter BE (1994) Stability of [3H] MK-801 binding sites following chronic ethanol consumption. Alcohol Clin Exp Res 18(4): 1004–1008
Trevisan L, Fitzgerald LW, Brose N, Gasic G, Heinemann SF, Duman RS, Nestler EJ (1994) Chronic ingestion of ethanol up-regulates NMDAR1 receptors subunit immunoreactivity in rat hippocampus. J Neurochem 62: 1635–1638
Tsai G, Gastfriend DR, Coyle JT (1995) The glutamatergic basis of human alcoholism. Am J Psychiatry 152(3): 332–340
Valverius P, Crabbe JC, Hoffman PL, Tabakoff B (1990) NMDA receptors in mice bred to be prone or resistant to ethanol withdrawal seizures. Eur J Pharmacol 184: 185–189
Verdoorn TA, Burnashev N, Monyer H, Seeburg PH, Sakmann B (1991) Structural determinants of ion flow through recombinant glutamate receptor channels. Science 252(5013): 1715–1718
Wang X, Lemos JR, Dayanithi G, Nordman JJ, Treistman SN (1991) Ethanol reduces vasopressin release by inhibiting calcium currents in nerve terminals. Brain Res 551: 338–341
Watkins JC, Oliverman HJ (1987) Agonists and antagonists for excitatory amino acid receptors. Trends Neurosci 10: 265–272
Weaver MS, Lee Y-H, Morris JL, Randall PK, Schallert T, Leslie SW (1993) Effects of in vitro ethanol and fetal ethanol exposure on glutathione stimulation of N-methyl-D-aspartate receptor function. Alcohol Clin Exp Res 17: 643–650
Weight FF, Peoples RW, Wright JM, Li C, Aguayo LG, Lovinger DM, White G (1993) Neurotransmitter-gated ion channels as molecular site of alcohol action. In: Alling C, Diamond I, Leslie SW, Sun GY, Wood WG (eds) Alcohol, cell membranes, and signal transduction in brain. Plenum, New York, pp 107–122
Wessinger WD, Balster RL (1987) Interactions between phencyclidine and central nervous system depressants evaluated in mice and rats. Pharmacol Biochem Behav 27: 323–332
Westbrook GL (1994) Glutamate receptor update. Curr Opin Neurobiol 4(3): 337–346
White G, Lovinger DM, Grant KA (1990) Ethanol (EtOH) inhibition of NMDA-activated ion current is not altered after chronic exposure of rats or neurons in culture. Alcohol Clin Exp Res 14(2): 352
Willetts J, Balster RL, Leander JD (1990) The behavioral pharmacology of NMDA receptor antagonists. Trends Pharmacol Sci 11(10): 423–428
Williams K (1993) Ifenprodil discriminates subtypes of the N-methyl-D-aspartate receptor: selectivity and mechanisms at recombinant heteromeric receptors. Mol Pharmacol 44: 851–859
Williams K, Russell SL, Shen YM, Molinoff PB (1993) Developmental switch in the expression of NMDA receptors occurs in vivo and in vitro. Neuron 10: 267–278
Wong EHF, Kemp JA (1991) Sites for antagonism on the N-methyl-D-aspartate receptor channel complex. Ann Rev Pharmacol Toxicol 31: 401–425
Wong EHF, Kemp J, Priestley T, Knight AR, Woodrugg GN, Iversen LL (1986) The anticonvulsant MK-801 is a potent N-methyl-D-aspartate antagonist. Proc Natl Acad Sci USA 83: 7104–7108
Wood SC, Hill WA, Miller KW (1993) Cycloalkanemethanols discriminate between volume- and length-dependent loss of activity of alkanols at the Torpedo nicotinic acetylcholine receptor. Mol Pharmacol 44(6): 1219–1226
Woodward JJ (1994) A comparison of the effects of ethanol and the competitive glycine antagonist 7-chlorokynurenic acid on N-methyl-D-aspartic acid-induced neurotransmitter release from rat hippocampal slices. J Neurochem 62(3): 987–991
Woodward JJ, Gonzales RA (1990) Ethanol inhibition of N-methyl-D-aspartate-stimulated endogenous dopamine release from rat striatal slices: reversal by glycine. J Neurochem 54: 712–715
Wu PH, Mihic SJ, Liu JF, Le AD, Kalant H (1993) Blockade of chronic tolerance to ethanol by the NMDA antagonist, (+)-MK-801. Eur J Pharmacol 231(2): 157–164
Zeise ML, Kasparov S, Capogna M, Zieglgansberger W (1993) Acamprosate (calciumacetylhomotaurinate) decreases postsynaptic potentials in the rat neocortex: possible involvement of excitatory amino acid receptors. Eur J Pharmacol 231(1): 47–52
Zhong J, Russell SL, Pritchett DB, Molinoff PB, Williams K (1994) Expression of mRNAs encoding subunits of the N-methyl-D-aspartate receptor in cultured cortical neurons. Mol Pharmacol 45: 846–853

The Neurobiology of Craving: Potential Mechanisms for Acamprosate

J. Littleton[1], M. al Qatari[1], and H. Little[2]

Introduction

There now seems no doubt that acamprosate is effective at reducing relapse into drinking in detoxified alcoholic patients (Lhuintre et al. 1985; Hillemand et al. 1984, 1989; Tran et al. 1990). However, the mechanism by which the drug achieves this effect is far from understood. Most conventional mechanisms of drugs that prevent relapse (see Liljequist and Borg 1993), such as making alcohol aversive or reducing the rewarding effects of the drug (Fig. 1), are not supported by the known pharmacology of acamprosate (see Littleton 1995). Self-reports from patients and clinical experience suggest that a major effect of acamprosate on relapse is to reduce the tendency for drinking episodes to escalate "out of control", and this is supported by increased indices of social stability in clinical trials of acamprosate (see Pelc et al. 1994; Lesch et al. 1994). This pattern suggests that acamprosate has a unique mechanism, and that its efficacy against relapse is a consequence of an ability to interrupt the process leading to loss of control in drinking behaviour. This might be described as an "anti-craving" action (see below, and Littleton 1995), but this leaves several important questions unanswered. First, how exactly are craving and loss of control related? Second, how could any drug interfere with such a mechanism (i.e. what is its chemical basis)? Third, how can we investigate such a mechanism? And fourth, does any of the known pharmacology of acamprosate support such a mechanism? This review attempts to answer some of these questions and suggests the approaches that we believe to be necessary to unravel the mystery of the mechanism of action of acamprosate.

How Are Craving and Loss of Control Related?

"Craving" is a common feature of most forms of drug dependence and provides a very common reason for relapse in detoxified drug abusers (see Wise 1988; Pickens and Johanson 1992). In alcoholism, subjective assessment of the strength of craving provides a good indicator of the likelihood of relapse (O'Connor et al. 1991), and therefore interfering with craving is an important

[1]Pharmacology Group, Kings College, Manresa Rd., London SW3 6LX, UK
[2]Psychology Department, University of Durham, Durham, UK

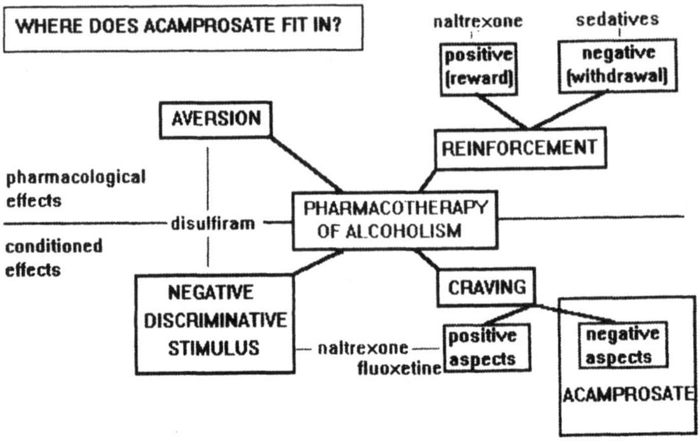

Fig. 1. *Current and potential pharmacotherapies for alcohol dependence.* The figure shows the different ways in which therapeutic agents are currently used to prevent alcohol relapse. These agents can alter the pharmacological effects of alcohol (*top half*) or the conditioned effects of the drug (*bottom half*). This separation is not absolute, and all agents probably affect both in some way. Thus the best known treatment, disulfiram, makes alcohol aversive (a pharmacological effect), but it prevents relapse by acting as a "negative discriminative stimulus": patients taking the drug know by experience (or by suggestion) that it will cause an aversive reaction if they drink alcohol (a conditioned effect). Disulfiram therefore is *useful* because it has a pharmacological effect, but its therapeutic *use* is based on the hope that this effect will never be seen! It is possible that agents which reduce the rewarding effects of alcohol (such as naltrexone?) also become negative discriminative stimuli. Acamprosate, together with some other new treatments, fits best into the category of an "anti-craving" agent. However, it is likely that there are differences in the types of craving that such drugs affect (see text), and this in turn may provide different indications for their use in recovering alcoholics

therapeutic goal (O'Brien et al. 1990; O'Brien 1994). Craving is associated with cues from the drug-taking past such as, in the case of alcohol, passing a familiar bar, seeing advertisements for alcoholic drinks, and being offered a drink at a party. Craving itself seems to consist of both positive and negative features (in much the same way that the reinforcing effects of drugs for drug-taking behaviour can be classified as positive or negative). Thus craving can be caused by *anticipation* of the drug *reward* (positive aspects) and/or by feelings of *anxiety and dysphoria* (negative aspects) that are perceived as capable of *amelioration* by taking the drug. Since both aspects of craving are initiated by cues associated with previous drinking behaviour (Childress et al. 1993; Glautier and Drummond 1994), they are undoubtedly attributable to "conditioning"; however, we suggest that the processes for positive and negative aspects are fundamentally different, and that this has important implications for their role in the initiation of relapse and for loss of control during relapse.

Conditioning and Craving

Operant conditioning plays a fundamental role in drug dependence. Thus drugs provide chemical rewards which contribute to the positive reinforcement to continue drug-taking behaviour. Additionally, when many drugs of dependence leave the brain, they cause anxiety and dysphoria, and these feelings provide negative reinforcements to re-take the drug. The combination of positive and negative reinforcements is what makes drugs addictive, and their strength is a measure of the addictive potential of a specific drug. However, classical, or pavlovian, conditioning also plays an important role when a drug is taken repeatedly (as it must be to cause dependence). Under these conditions the drug reward is repeatedly paired with the behaviour associated with its administration and with the environment in which the drug is usually taken. This means that these associated stimuli become conditioned to the drug reward and take on rewarding characteristics themselves as a result (e.g. Robinson and Berridge 1993; Childress et al. 1993). This simple association is probably sufficient to explain the positive aspects of drug craving (see below).

Positive Aspects of Craving

When an individual has repeatedly received the chemical reward that alcohol provides (relaxation, euphoria, excitement) as a consequence of drinking alcohol in similar environments (bars, restaurants etc.), classical conditioning is predicted to make him or her experience the same subjective feelings in response to these conditioned stimuli. Thus the cues associated with drinking, passing a bar, being offered a drink etc. should elicit anticipatory feelings similar to the positively reinforcing properties of the drug itself. The situation is exactly analogous to Pavlov's dogs, where the conditioned stimulus (the sound of a bell) was able to elicit the conditioned response (salivation) even in the absence of the unconditioned stimulus (food). Here the familiar bar elicits the anticipation of the alcohol reward even in the absence of the alcohol. It is quite easy to speculate that this is the basis for positive aspects of craving. An individual who anticipates the reward associated with the drug each time he or she encounters drug-related cues might well find it difficult to maintain abstinence. In the case of alcohol such cues are so widely distributed in our society that they would make it extremely difficult not to relapse into drinking. The positive aspects of craving are simple to understand and are a reasonable explanation for *initiation* of drinking behaviour. The negative aspects of withdrawal are less easy to understand, but they are at least as important because they appear to provide a better explanation for loss of control once a relapse into drinking has been initiated.

Negative Aspects of Craving

When drug administration is repeated frequently, an almost inevitable consequence is the development of drug tolerance. Among the mechanisms for this are adaptations within the central nervous system that oppose the effects of the drug (see Samson and Harris 1992). It is known that such adaptations in the brain can themselves become conditioned to associated stimuli, for example, in a direct parallel to Pavlov's experiments, when a centrally acting *drug*, such as apomorphine, is used as a stimulus for salivation (rather than food) what eventually becomes conditioned to the paired stimulus (the bell) is the opposing *adaptation* to the drug (see Steward et al. 1984). As a result, presenting the bell in the absence of the drug leads to the opposite effect, in this case a dry mouth resulting from reduced salivation. The cue provided by the bell has initiated opposing adaptation to the drug in the brain, but because the drug has not been presented, only the adaptation is observed. This rather subtle type of conditioning has been most clearly and most often demonstrated in the phenomenon of "environment-dependent tolerance" (see Siegel 1979) in which experimental animals and humans exhibit greatest tolerance to a drug in the environment in which it has been given, rather than in an environment not associated with the drug. The explanation is probably that the drug environment acts as a cue initiating the adaptive mechanism for the drug even before the drug has arrived in the brain. The "primed" brain is therefore able to better withstand the chemical assault caused by the drug when it does arrive, and the organism therefore demonstrates a greater degree of drug tolerance.

There is no doubt that drug adaptation can be conditioned, but what does it have to do with craving and loss of control in drinking behaviour? As a mechanism for negative aspects of craving, the explanation is fairly straightforward (see Siegel 1979; Steward et al. 1984). Exposure to a cue related to past drinking should set off adaptation in the brain designed to oppose the chemical effects of alcohol. If no alcohol reaches the brain despite the appropriate cue, the adaptation is not balanced by the drug. The consequence are feelings opposite to those normally caused by the drug – "opponent processes" in psychological jargon. In the case of alcohol (which causes relaxation, excitement and euphoria) these are anxiety, depression and dysphoria. The recovering alcoholic knows from past experience with the drug that these feelings will be rapidly reversed by drinking alcohol, and this contributes to his or her craving (see O'Brien 1994). This is a reasonable description of the negative aspects of craving (though the explanation may be wildly inaccurate!), and it is easy to see that this may contribute to initiation of relapse. However, why should it have anything to do with loss of control once relapse has occurred?

Craving and Loss of Control

Probably one of the most effective cues for craving is being offered a drink, since this has previously almost always preceded drinking behaviour and is thus very strongly associated with this. Let us speculate on how this cue may lead first to craving, then to relapse, and then to loss of control over drinking behaviour. Because of its strong associations with alcohol the presentation of this cue sets off positive feelings of anticipation of the alcohol reward, mixed with negative feelings of anxiety and depression that will be overcome by drinking alcohol. The individual succumbs to the resulting craving and initiates drinking behaviour. This *itself* acts as a cue, as does the subsequent arrival of alcohol in the mouth, the stomach, the circulation, and finally the brain. In fact, all of these provide successive cues of increasing immediacy for the effects of alcohol on the brain, and for the adaptation to these effects. They all make craving worse! In addition, because it has been primed to adapt to alcohol by all these cues, the brain is "ahead of the game". It is very difficult for the individual to "catch up" with the adaptation to alcohol in the brain without drinking faster and faster, but if he or she tries this approach, the increasing physiological and mental effects of alcohol act as additional cues for adaptation. This can be viewed as the psychological and neurochemical equivalent of a treadmill, the faster you drink the faster you need to drink. If this is a true representation of the situation it certainly helps explain loss of control. "One drink, one drunk!" as Alcoholics Anonymous warns its members.

Craving: Conclusions

The above explanations are undoubtedly oversimplified, and may be quite wrong. There are many other more sophisticated variations on these (e.g. Modell et al. 1992; Robinson and Berridge 1993) Most research workers would accept that craving is a very complex aspect of drug dependence, but some even doubt its existence. We make no apologies for out attempts to explain craving in simple mechanistic terms because without such hypotheses we could not investigate useful drugs such as acamprosate. The framework developed above suggests that positive aspects of craving might be prevented by drugs that interfere with the chemical rewarding effects of abused drugs (see Fig. 1). Inhibition of dopamine release or receptor activation would be a possibility, though there are no currently used examples. Inhibition of opioid receptors would be another, and naltrexone, which has recently been accepted as a therapy that reduces alcoholic relapse, may work in this way (Volpicelli et al. 1992). Finally, serotonin uptake inhibitors such as fluoxetine may inhibit anticipatory or "appetitive" behaviour and have been found to be useful in preventing relapse (e.g. Gerra et al. 1992). Thus, for the positive aspects of craving we have some idea of the transmitter systems involved, but this does not help to understand acamprosate, which appears to affect none of these. So what are the potential chemical mechanisms for the negative aspects of craving?

Chemical Mechanisms for the Negative Aspects of Craving

There has been an explosion of research into the adaptations that oppose the effects of alcohol in the brains of animals (see Samson and Harris 1992). To date, much of this supports at least three types of adaptation, involving the receptors for the two major neurotransmitters in the mammalian brain (the amino acids, GABA and glutamate) and a subclass of calcium channels (proteins that have a major influence on neuronal excitability). In all cases these adaptations are thought to oppose the effects of alcohol, and in all cases they are also suggested to play a role in the alcohol withdrawal syndrome as well as contributing to alcohol tolerance (see Samson and Harris 1992). Since the negative aspects of craving (anxiety, depression, dysphoria) strongly resemble the "early minor signs" of alcohol withdrawal, it is possible that true withdrawal and the conditioned "pseudo-withdrawal" of craving share similar mechanisms.

True Withdrawal and Pseudo-withdrawal

The chemical basis for true alcohol withdrawal is thought to be that adaptations which have been induced in the brain by the long-term presence of alcohol are exposed by removal of the drug; these adaptations then cause the functional changes that make up the withdrawal syndrome (Samson and Harris 1992; Littleton and Little 1994). The sequence of events can be represented as a cartoon see-saw (Fig. 2) in which withdrawal occurs because of a chemical "overbalance" when the drug leaves the brain. This overbalance (and thus the withdrawal signs that it causes) continue until the adaptation can be removed from the brain (Fig. 2). This explanation for withdrawal, an opposing adaptation that is not balanced by the presence of the drug, is therefore almost identical to our previous explanation of the negative aspects of craving. Figure 3 illustrates the principles behind craving using the same see-saw analogy of Fig. 2, and this should highlight the similarities. In craving, the conditioned adaptation is unbalanced because the drug has not been administered; in withdrawal, the unconditioned adaptation is unbalanced because the drug has left the brain. However, although the concepts, and their consequences, are very similar, this does not mean that the mechanisms involved are identical.

Differences Between Withdrawal and Craving

The adaptations that lead to true alcohol withdrawal seem to require prolonged periods of alcohol exposure, both for their institution and for their removal (see Samson and Harris 1992). The models in which they are studied utilise continuous exposure of animals to high concentrations of alcohol for at least several days. These conditions are necessary to induce an observable withdrawal syndrome in laboratory animals, and in man. They also produce changes in gene expression of key membrane proteins on nerves (receptors and ion channels) that persist for many hours after removal of alcohol from the system, and it is these kinds of long-term adaptations that are thought to underlie the signs of withdrawal (see Littleton and Little 1994). In fact, it is a prerequisite for adaptations that cause withdrawal that they are *semi-permanent.* They must persist after alcohol has left the brain in order to cause the chemical "overbalance" that leads to withdrawal. This semi-permanence is also the reason why we know so much about these changes; they persist after death, and we can therefore use sophisticated neurochemical techniques on the post-mortem brain to identify the changes associated with alcohol administration and withdrawal. However, although there has been a huge basic research effort in uncovering these alcohol-induced adaptations, they are probably completely

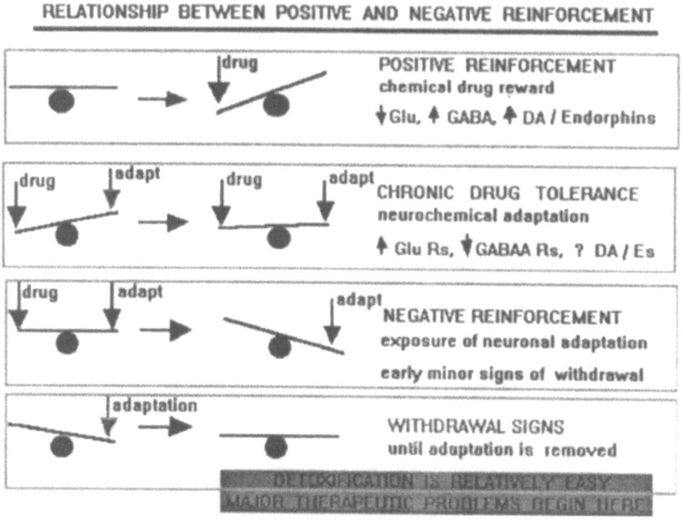

Fig. 2. *Cartoon, showing the development of adaptations to alcohol in the brain and its relationship to tolerance and withdrawal.* The figure shows brain activity depicted as a see-saw, which is "unbalanced" towards "relaxation" etc. by the acute effect of alcohol (its chemical rewarding effect). As the presence of alcohol is maintained for a period of several days, opposing adaptive responses are gradually induced in the brain which eventually balance the effect of alcohol. The brain then performs relatively normally even while alcohol is still present (tolerance). However, if alcohol is then rapidly removed from the brain (withdrawal) the adaptation is no longer balanced by the drug, and the system "overbalances" into excitation. The early consequences of this, anxiety and dysphoria, are thought to play major roles in the negative reinforcements for drinking behaviour. These and other functional consequences of the adaptation to alcohol make up the "withdrawal syndrome", which continues until the adaptation to alcohol is removed by the brain. Treating the signs of withdrawal associated with the overbalance toward excitation is relatively easy; sedatives and tranquillisers can cover the withdrawal syndrome and allow relatively symptom-free detoxification. The main therapeutic problem is to maintain abstinence once detoxification is complete, and this probably requires drugs that interfere with the ability of conditioned stimuli to initiate drinking behaviour

inappropriate as *conditioned* adaptations to the drug leading to pseudo-withdrawal. It could be argued that this is a therapeutically more important research goal, and investigating mechanisms for drugs such as acamprosate may lead us closer to this (see below).

In contrast to true withdrawal, the adaptations that produce conditioned pseudo-withdrawal must, almost by definition, be very *rapid*. They are designed to oppose drug effects that are "expected" in the brain almost immediately, and changes such as those due to altered gene expression are probably much too slow to be considered for this role. In addition, in order for the adaptations responsible to be *conditioned* by the drug-taking behaviour and environment the absolute requirement is that drug administrations must be discrete and *frequent*. In contrast, the regime of alcohol that best produces true withdrawal signs is a *continuous* administration, though the severity of withdrawal is increased if administrations are repeated (Becker 1994).

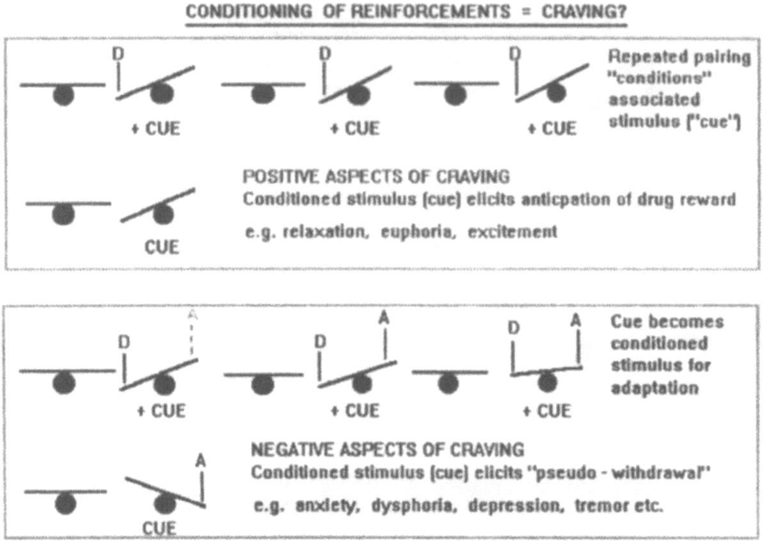

Fig. 3. *How conditioning of positive and negative reinforcing effects of alcohol may underlie craving. Top half,* the early stages of alcohol use in which the drug is taken repeatedly in association with a specific cue (the interior of a neighbourhood bar, for example). As the chemical rewarding effect of the drug (the unbalancing of the brain see-saw toward relaxation and intoxication) is repeatedly "paired" with the cue, this becomes a conditioned stimulus for the same chemical effects that the drug produces. At this stage (theoretically) the individual could walk into the bar and begin to anticipate relaxation even before drinking. The cue (the conditioned stimulus) has become capable of eliciting the chemical response, even in the absence of the unconditioned stimulus (the drug). *Bottom half,* the situation later in the drinking history. As the individual repeatedly drinks in the bar, opposing adaptive responses to the drug are induced in the brain. Some of these may always be present (the kind that lead to dependence and true withdrawal), but some may be short-term responses, produced "to order" as the drug appears in the brain each day. The latter type are always "paired" with the environment of the bar, and therefore as they become stronger and stronger, gradually limiting the chemical effect of the drug on the brain see-saw, the environment becomes a conditioned stimulus for the adaptations. Once this stage is reached, simply walking into the bar is sufficient to initiate the adaptive response to alcohol, this constitutes "environment-dependent" tolerance. However, if the individual now walks into the bar but does not drink alcohol, the adaptation is unopposed and "overbalances" the brain see-saw in the opposite direction. This causes pseudo-withdrawal, which, we suggest, constitutes a major negative aspect of craving

If the mechanisms leading to true alcohol withdrawal are too slow to be candidates for the pseudo-withdrawal of craving, then what are the possibilities? Rapid responses of the central nervous system are far more likely to be caused by alterations in neuronal electrical activity and transmitter release rather than by alterations in receptor proteins or ion channels. However, with a bewildering complexity of neuronal pathways and a huge variety of neurotransmitter candidates to chose from, this is not immediately helpful. Nevertheless, we do have some clues, both from our knowledge of the acute mechanisms of action of alcohol and from the systems which show adaptations leading to true alcohol withdrawal. After all, since some of the consequences of the true and pseudo-withdrawal are similar, it is possible that the same systems are involved, even if the mechanisms differ.

Neurotransmitter Systems and Negative Aspects of Craving

In general terms, the neurochemical basis of alcohol withdrawal can be characterised as an increase in neuronal excitability associated with reduced inhibition via the GABAergic system and increased excitation via the glutamatergic system (see Samson and Harris 1992). The increased excitation may be further enhanced by the alcohol-induced increase in calcium channel proteins on nerves (see Littleton and Little 1994). These changes are able to account for many of the psychological and physical signs of withdrawal, with the exception of dysphoria; this sign may be explained by a reduction in dopamine release in forebrain limbic areas by analogy to the effects seen on opiate withdrawal (Diana et al. 1995), but this has not yet been much studied for alcohol.

Since the same signs characterise the pseudo-withdrawal of craving, attempts to explain these have centered on alterations in the transmitters GABA, glutamate and dopamine. Some evidence in support is supplied by experiments which implicate both GABA and glutamate in the nucleus accumbens in ethanol self-administration in rats (Rassnick et al. 1992). If a conditioned alteration in neuronal activity and transmitter release is the explanation for negative aspects of craving, we would predict that the conditioned stimuli should reduce GABA and dopamine release, and increase glutamate release. At present there is no evidence for or against any of these, and there are several other possibilities. Our own preference is for an increase in glutamate release (or for an increase in release of the other major excitatory amino acid transmitter, aspartate). This is only because it is easier to imagine a stimulus provoking an increase in neuronal activity rather than a reduction, and it is certainly easier to *measure* an increase in transmitter release in the brain in vivo rather than a reduction!

Withdrawal and Craving: Conclusions

This section has been very speculative, but there is really no alternative. Basic neurochemical research has made no concerted attempt to investigate psychological aspects of dependence other than those associated with drug *rewards* before. Indeed, the concepts outlined above are foreign to most pharmacologists (which is probably why we have made such a poor attempt at explaining them), and this has been more an exercise in formulating hypotheses than proposing explanations. In order to proceed with our discussion of how acamprosate might work we assume that a major form of conditioned adaptation is that glutamate and/or aspartate release is increased in some brain areas when conditioned stimuli associated with alcohol self-administration are encountered. The release of these transmitters is designed to increase the level of neuronal excitation so that this "balances" the depressant effect of alcohol as soon as the drug reaches the brain. The relevance to craving is, of course, that the conditioned excitation is unopposed if alcohol does *not* reach the brain, and this causes some of the negative aspects of craving that we describe as "pseudo-withdrawal". This seems to us to be a reasonable hypothesis, but, as with all hypotheses, it is of little use unless it is testable. Unfortunately, in order to achieve this, it is necessary to invent almost a whole new branch of pharmacological research.

How Can We Investigate Anti-craving Drugs?

There are no animal models for drug self-administration that are universally accepted though there are some principles that are agreed. In the case of alcohol, which can be given orally, it is common to provide a choice of drinking water or alcohol solution. Since laboratory rodents do not normally drink sufficient alcohol to produce pharmacological effects, it is usual to precede the test period with some procedure designed to increase this, adding a sweetener to the alcohol-containing solution, for example, or inducing some degree of physical dependence by forced administration of alcohol before the animals are given a free choice. Such methods can undoubtedly be used as screening procedures to obtain data on potential therapeutic agents (see below), but they are not well suited to assessing effects on *relapse* into alcohol use after detoxification, which is the major therapeutic problem. They are certainly unsuitable for investigating subtle neurochemical mechanisms for conditioning related to craving, and this is what is necessary here.

Requirements for a Model

In order for conditioning to occur the stimuli required to be conditioned must be presented *repeatedly*. In this case, alcohol and the stimuli to be conditioned (a specific environment?) must therefore be presented together sufficiently often for them to become associated. Additionally, for observable signs of withdrawal to be produced, a period of a few days of alcohol exposure is probably necessary, and for immediate signs of withdrawal to dissipate between exposures a period of about 24 h is necessary (all figures are for laboratory rodents). We use alcohol inhalation as our method of exposure to the drug because of our familiarity with the procedure and because it can be standardised between animals, but other methods could be equally appropriate. What we should aim for is therefore (perhaps!) repeated (say, six) alcohol exposures to the point of mild intoxication for 3–4 days, interspersed with 1-day withdrawal periods. Alcohol exposures should be in a specific environment and withdrawal in a quite different environment (so that the stress of withdrawal does not become associated with the alcohol-related environment). Under these conditions it is predicted that the environment in which the animals repeatedly receive alcohol should become a conditioned stimulus for adaptation to alcohol in the brain. After the animals have been detoxified a final time, exposure to the alcohol-related environment *alone* (or perhaps with a brief exposure to a low concentration of alcohol?) should elicit the adaptation and cause conditioned pseudo-withdrawal. This in turn can be used to test the effects of drugs on this negative aspect of craving (if this is a correct assumption), and the model can certainly be used to investigate the neurochemical mechanisms for these phenomena. However, deciding exactly what to measure is still a problem.

Behavioural and Physiological Measures of Craving

Even in clinical experiments it is hard to decide what constitute appropriate measures of craving (see Rosenhow et al. 1990; Robbins and Ehrman 1992). For animals it is considerably more difficult because *introspective* assessments (in many ways the most important) are impossible; you cannot ask a rat how much it needs a drink! We are therefore thrown back on observation, but without much idea of what exactly we are looking for. Again, we must improvise, and since we have characterised negative aspects of craving as pseudo-withdrawal we chose our measures from those that have been found useful in true withdrawal in rodents, together with other measures that should intuitively be important in craving.

Anxiety

The early signs of true drug withdrawal in humans include anxiety, and this is one of the main negative aspects of craving cited in clinical studies (e.g. Swift and Stout 1992; Glautier and Drummond 1994). Measures of anxiety (plus maze, light/dark box, open-field exploration, acoustic startle response) have also been used in animal models of true alcohol withdrawal (e.g. File et al. 1993). Measures of anxiety are therefore imperative here, but many are precluded by the necessity of testing for anxiety in the *specific environment* associated with alcohol administration. Of the measures listed above only the acoustic startle response is appropriate, and this, together with close observation, for example, of social interaction between animals, is probably the best choice. Animals conditioned and then exposed to the alcohol-related environment in the absence of alcohol are predicted to show a higher level of anxiety than animals exposed to a neutral environment (or, as a control, those exposed to the environment associated with withdrawal).

Drug-Seeking Behaviour

The most relevant sign of craving related to initiation of relapse is the observation of drug-seeking behaviour; however, in a *forced* alcohol administration paradigm, such as inhalation, animals would never learn to associate alcohol ingestion with relief of withdrawal. One could not therefore expect them to show increased alcohol-seeking during pseudo-withdrawal. The dilemma might be resolved by allowing free-choice access to alcohol for several days before forced alcohol administration, and then throughout all alcohol exposure and withdrawal periods. Under these conditions we have previously been able to induce increases in alcohol consumption during true withdrawal. The prediction here is that exposure to the alcohol-related environment in the absence of alcohol should induce pseudo-withdrawal, and this should cause an increase in voluntary alcohol consumption.

Drug Self-Administration

At first glance this is identical to the measures above; however if conditioned adaptation precipitates "loss of control" drinking, this may be qualitatively different from drinking under other circumstances. For example, alcohol intake may be very great in the early stages of pseudo-withdrawal and then slacken as intoxication occurs. Also, the pressure to *maintain* alcohol intake over 24 h may be less than in true withdrawal as the adaptation causing pseudo-withdrawal subsides more rapidly. The pattern of voluntary alcohol consumption may be different in the conditioned model, and this should not be ignored.

Physical and Autonomic Signs

Both craving (Glautier and Drummond 1994) and the early minor signs of true alcohol withdrawal in man are associated with tremors and shakes, and to a certain extent these can be measured in laboratory rodents. In addition, true alcohol withdrawal in mice is associated with mild seizures, characterised as "convulsions on handling" which are easy to score by a trained observer (e.g. see Littleton and Little 1994). Whether or not these are directly relevant to any aspect of craving is uncertain, but they *are* thought to represent an effect of opposing adaptation to alcohol in the brain. Their great advantage here is that they are a standard, accepted, and robust physical measure of alcohol withdrawal. They are predicted to be increased by exposure to the conditioned stimulus, i.e. the environment associated with alcohol exposure, in the absence of ethanol.

Autonomic signs are thought by some to be of considerable importance in craving for stimulants and opiates (Steward et al. 1984), but there is some controversy over the importance of autonomic signs in alcohol craving (see McCusker and Brown 1995). Nevertheless, true alcohol withdrawal in man is associated with signs of increased activity of the sympathetic nervous system, piloerection, sweating and increased heart rate. Of these, piloerection can be observed in rodents and should be included. Other measurable autonomic signs, including alterations in body temperature should also be considered.

Biochemical Measures of Craving

There are two reasons for seeking biochemical signs in conditioned pseudo-withdrawal. One is to establish quantifiable measures to confirm and underscore the subjective observations of behavioural change, and the other is to investigate the mechanism for the changes observed.

Peripheral Measures of Stress

Measures of stress associated with true withdrawal include increased circulating catecholamines, glucocorticoids, free fatty acids and triglycerides. All of these are potential measures in these studies. They all suffer from the disadvantage that collection of blood from small rodents is itself a very stressful procedure. This is probably less important in true withdrawal (which is probably highly stressful and prolonged) than it may be for conditioned pseudo-withdrawal (which may be briefer and more subtle). Nevertheless, measurements of this type should be attempted.

Immediate Early Gene Expression

True alcohol withdrawal is associated with increased expression of the immediate early gene, c-*fos*, in a specific distribution in the rodent brain (Morgan et al. 1992). This gene is in fact a relatively non-specific marker for neuronal excitation and is increased by stress and by release of excitatory amino acids in the brain. Investigating whether increased c-Fos protein expression is associated with presentation of the conditioned environment will therefore help to confirm whether pseudo-withdrawal occurs as a result of changes in the *brain*. However, it goes very much further than that. The distribution of c-Fos in conditioned pseudo-withdrawal can be compared with that in true withdrawal to assess, whether the same neuronal systems are involved. The distribution of c-Fos also allows us to predict which precise areas of the brain are likely to yield conditioned alterations in transmitter release. Indeed by using selective inhibitors (e.g. glutamate receptor antagonists) we can assess which transmitters are likely to be involved in the response. Finally, the expression of c-Fos on exposure to the conditioned environment can itself be used as the response to test whether agents such as acamprosate directly affect the *neuronal* processes causing craving.

Neurotransmitter Release

The only way that alterations in transmitter release can be followed during exposure to the conditioned environment would be by brain perfusion dialysis (or electrochemical detection with implanted probes) in conscious animals.

This would be difficult and cannot be justified in the absence of preliminary data that the phenomenon exists in laboratory animals, and that specific brain areas and transmitters are implicated (e.g. by c-Fos experiments as above). Once these have been accomplished measurements of transmitter release in vivo becomes a priority and is the only way in which final mechanisms for these phenomena can be established.

Models for Craving: Conclusions

We have only recently recognised that models for this type of craving are necessary (the stimulus was the necessity of investigating the mechanism of action of drugs such as acamprosate), and we have therefore not made substantial progress toward establishing the exact experimental conditions required. Nevertheless, our experience of animal models for true alcohol withdrawal (which took many years to develop) make us confident of eventual success. Even the process of discussion and debate has been useful; it has led to the suggestion that acamprosate is an agent that uniquely suppresses conditioned pseudo-withdrawal.

How Does Acamprosate Fit into These Concepts?

Acamprosate is acetylhomotaurine, a simple derivative of a simple amino acid, taurine. Historically, it was developed from taurine because this is a common ingredient of several Oriental medicines, claimed to be of use as "anti-craving" agents in drug dependence. Acamprosate has close similarities with some of the naturally occurring excitatory amino acids (such as glutamate, aspartate and homocysteic acid) as well as naturally occurring inhibitory amino acids (GABA and taurine). These structural similarities provide little help in identifying its mechanism of action, except to suggest that amino acid transmitters are those most likely to be affected by the drug (see Littleton 1995). Since the pharmacology of acamprosate has recently been reviewed by one of us (Littleton 1995) the following sections are only summaries.

Behavioural Effects of Acamprosate

Acamprosate is not sedative and does not potentiate the sedative effects of ethanol (Le Magnen et al. 1987b). Its activity in more sophisticated behavioural tests (such as for anxiolytic or antidepressant activity) is unknown. It appears to have no abuse potential based on tests of reinforcing and discriminative stimulus properties (Grant and Woolverton 1989). All the available evidence suggests that it is without significant behavioural effects unless it is tested against alcohol dependence (see below). Whether these effects on alcohol can be generalised to other drug dependence states is unknown (but is an important question).

Drug Self-Administration

Acamprosate reduces self-administration of alcohol by rodents in a variety of paradigms (Boismare et al. 1984; Le Magnen et al. 1987a; Gewiss et al. 1991). It appears to be most effective in models in which prior forced administration of alcohol has induced some degree of dependence (e.g. Le Magnen et al. 1987). This is compatible with a reduction in the negatively reinforcing effects of alcohol withdrawal (and with an anti-craving action for the drug).

Physical Signs of Withdrawal

Acamprosate is a fairly weak inhibitor of the physical signs of withdrawal from alcohol (see Littleton 1985). These of course are less relevant to craving than early minor signs such as anxiety, but these do not appear to have been investigated.

Biochemical Effects of Acamprosate

Apart from its similarity to amino acids the structure of acamprosate offers few clues as to its mechanism. The drug certainly shows no resemblance to alcohol, and it does not interfere with alcohol metabolism at the alcohol or aldehyde dehydrogenase steps. It is very unlikely that it either substitutes for alcohol, or that is makes alcohol aversive by altering its metabolism.

Immediate Early Gene Expression

Just as it is a weak inhibitor of the physical signs of true alcohol withdrawal so is acamprosate a weak inhibitor of the increased c-Fos expression associated with withdrawal (Bouchenafa et al. 1994). In fact, this effect is rather equivocal because acamprosate seems to reduce the intensity of expression rather than reducing the number of neurons showing c-Fos expression, and this makes quantitation extremely difficult. Nevertheless, this is compatible with effects on pseudo-withdrawal, and we are currently attempting to measure the effects of acamprosate on conditioned c-Fos expression in rodent brain.

Effects on Neurotransmitter Receptor Activation

Electrophysiologically, acamprosate reduces neuronal hyper-excitation in brain in vivo when this is caused by activation of excitatory amino acid receptors (Zeise et al. 1990, 1993). It appears to have little or no effect on inhibition induced by GABA, at least in the cortical neurones studied (Zeise et al. 1993). The mechanism of inhibition of excitation is unknown, and attempts to find related effects on excitatory amino acids in other systems, for example, cell cultures, have not always been successful (unpublished). The exception is a report from our laboratory that acamprosate reduces effects of excitatory amino acids on bovine adrenal cells (Bouchenala et al. 1990). However, the excitatory amino acid (glutamate) receptors in these cells differ from those on central neurones, making the finding of doubtful relevance to effects of acamprosate in the brain. The mechanism of these inhibitory effects on excitatory amino acid induced responses is unlikely to be directly glutamate receptor mediated because acamprosate is incapable of displacing a variety of radioligands for excitatory amino acid receptors from adrenal cell or neuronal membranes (unpublished). Acamprosate presumably does have its own receptors; however, because saturable, specific binding to brain membranes has been reported (Daoust et al. 1994).

A potential explanation for the electrophysiological findings in brain is that acamprosate decreases excitatory mechanisms "downstream" of excitatory amino acid receptor activation, and indeed calcium current "spiking" seems most affected by the drug (Zeise et al. 1993). This prompted us to investigate effects of acamprosate on binding of the calcium channel ligand isradipine to brain membranes (al Qatari and Littleton 1995). The results show that acamprosate is a potent displacer of [^{3}H]isradipine, but only when this ligand binds to a relatively low-affinity site (*c.*10–20 n*M*) rather than the conventional calcium channel protein site (*c.*0.5 n*M* affinity). This *suggests* that some type of calcium channel is affected by acamprosate, but more experiments are clearly necessary to establish this.

Effects on Neurotransmitter Release

Experiments to assess the effects of acamprosate on neurotransmitter release are in their infancy. It has been reported that in combination with ethanol the drug increases taurine release from rodent brain in vivo (Dahchour et al. 1994), and this is potentially a very important finding. Taurine is a naturally occurring inhibitory amino acid, and its release could reduce effects of the excitatory amino acids, whether released in response to alcohol withdrawal or in response to conditioned pseudo-withdrawal. When more preliminary data in the latter situation have been obtained, this could become an important possibility for investigation.

Acamprosate Mechanisms: Conclusions

We do not know how acamprosate works. From a process of exclusion we are left with an anti-craving mechanism for the drug, and this is compatible with its history, with subjective reports and with clinical experience. In so far as we have any basic pharmacological knowledge which is relevant to such an action, this too supports the proposal. The exact mechanism can only be guessed at, but acamprosate does seem to reduce states of neuronal hyperexcitability associated with activation of excitatory amino acid receptors. All this points to an inhibition of negative aspects of craving as the most plausible explanation for its clinical efficacy. All we have to do now is prove this!

What Needs to Be Done to Establish an Anti-craving Mechanism

Neither clinical research nor basic research alone can establish unequivocally the mechanism of action of acamprosate, or indeed any of its competitors or successors. There is an absolute need for a partnership between clinical and basic science in this area of therapeutics. Unfortunately, these agents belong to an entirely new class of drug, and the techniques required to investigate their mechanisms in either branch of medical science hardly exist. The following are some rather naive suggestions as a framework for more detailed discussion.

Clinical Research

Although attempts are beginning to characterise the conditions under which acamprosate is effective (e.g. Gerra et al. 1992; Poldrugo et al. 1994), this is not yet sufficient to help establish a mechanism. Clinically, the next step must be a detailed psychological evaluation of the subjective reasons why acamprosate is effective in those patients who do benefit from the drug. Do they truly control their drinking more easily? Are indices of craving reduced in the presence of alcohol-related cues? Are the patients who respond to acamprosate those in whom negative aspects of craving are particularly severe, whereas those who do not respond have other reasons for their drinking being out of control? These types of research (based on questionnaires and interviews) would be valuably supplemented by clinical experiments, in which psychological and physiological indices of stress are measured in response to selected cues while receiving acamprosate or placebo. There are undeniable technical and ethical problems with such experiments (see Robbins and Ehrman 1992), but they are essential to assess any anti-craving mechanism in man.

Basic Research

We have already given our own view of appropriate experiments in which to model the specific type of craving that we call conditioned pseudo-withdrawal. However, we recognise this as a very narrow and selective approach (for example, see Wise 1988). What is really needed from basic researchers in the drug dependence field is a willingness to step outside the "safe" areas of tolerance and physical dependence, where easily measurable parameters yield definitive results and to consider other, potentially more important problems. An example is given by attempts to induce conditioned withdrawal from opiates (Baldwin and Koob 1993). "Listening" to acamprosate (to borrow a phrase) has given us the stimulus to think more carefully about the therapeutic approaches to alcohol dependence that may be valuable in the future. There is little doubt that anti-craving drugs are a more important goal than improving drugs for detoxification (which is all that might be expected from work on physical dependence and withdrawal). Before acamprosate there was little positive evidence that a basic science approach to craving would ever bear therapeutic fruit. Those days are past.

Conclusion

Acamprosate appears to be a novel drug that is useful in preventing relapse in weaned alcoholics without having any of the mechanisms previously associated with such drugs. We have presented evidence that acamprosate is an anti-craving drug which might be particularly effective against the type of craving that we have called "conditioned pseudo-withdrawal". It will be a considerable challenge to establish whether this suggestion is correct but this is not the only point of this review. What we have tried to do is to establish that even in animal experiments there are ways to investigate in animals something as subtle and nebulous as craving, using standard behavioural and neurochemical techniques. We may be quite wrong in our explanations, and the approach we have outlined may prove to be futile, but at least we have recognised that here is an important aspect of the pharmacology of alcohol that has hitherto been ignored.

References

Al Qatari M, Littleton JM (1995) Acamprosate potently displaces [3H]isradipine from rat brain membranes. Alcohol Alcohol 30: 551 (10.16)

Baldwin HA, Koob GF (1993) Rapid induction of conditioned opiate withdrawal in the rat. Neuropsychopharmacology 8: 15–21

Becker HC (1994) Positive relationship between the number of prior ethanol withdrawal episodes and the severity of subsequent withdrawal seizures. Psychopharmacology 116: 26–32

Boismare F, Daoust M, Moore N, Saligaut C, Lhuintre JP, Chretien P, Durlach J (1984) A homotaurine derivative reduces the voluntary intake of ethanol of rats: are cerebral GABA receptors involved? Pharmacol Biochem Behav 21: 787–789

Bouchenafa O, Cwynarski K, Littleton JM (1990) Interactions between excitatory amino acids and AOTAL in a cell culture model of ethanol dependence. Alcohol Clin Exp Res 14: 312

Bouchenafa O, Davies R, Littleton JM (1994) Immunocytochemical localisation of c-fos expression in rat brain during ethanol withdrawal. Alcohol Clin Exp Res 18: 39A

Childress AR, Hole AV, Ehrman RN, Robbins SJ, McLellan AT, O'Brien CP (1993) Cue reactivity and cue reactivity interventions in drug dependence. NIDA Res Monogr 137: 73–95

Dahchour A, Quertemont E, De Witte P (1994) Acute ethanol increases taurine, but neither GABA nor glutamate in the nucleus accumbens: a microdialysis study in the male rat. Pflugers Arch Eur J Physiol 427: 3–4

Daoust M, Legrand E, Durbin P (1994) Binding characteristics of [3H]acamprosate to neuronal membrane preparations. Alcohol Clin Exp Res 18: 33A

Diana M, Pistis M, Muntoni A, Gessa G (1995) Profound decrease of mesolimbic dopaminergic neuronal activity in morphine withdrawn rats. J Pharmacol Exp Ther 272: 781–785

File SE, Andrews N, Al-Farhan M (1993) Anxiogenic responses of rats on withdrawal from chronic ethanol treatment: effects of tianeptine. Alcohol Alcohol 28: 281–286

Gerra G, Caccavari R, Delsignore R, Bocchi R, Fertonani G, Passeri M (1992) Effects of fluoxetine and calcium acetylhomotaurinate on alcohol intake in familial and nonfamilial alcoholic patients. Curr Ther Clin Exp 52: 291–295

Gewiss M, Heidbreder C, Opsomer L, Durbin P, Dewitte P (1991) Acamprosate and diazepam differentially modulate alcohol-induced behavioural and cortical alterations in rats following chronic inhalation of alcohol vapour. Alcohol Alcohol 26: 129–137

Glautier S, Drummond DC (1994) Alcohol dependence and cue reactivity. J Stud Alcohol 55: 224–229

Grant KA, Woolverton D (1989) Reinforcing and discriminative stimulus effects of calcium-acetyl homotaurine in animals. Pharmacol Biochem Behav 32: 607–611

Hillemand B, Lhuintre JP, Boismare F et al (1984) Premier-essai favorable du N-bis-acetylhomotaurinate du calcium dans la traitement de l'aloolo-dependant. Rev Alcool 30: 204–212

Hillemond B, Lhiuntre JP, Steru L, Boismare F, Daoust M, Moore N et al (1989) Essai therapeutique multicentrique du N-bisacetyl-homotaurinate de calcium dans la traitement de alocoolo-dependant. Rev Alcool 34: 9–28

Le Magnen J, Tran G, Durlach J, Martin C (1987a) Dose-dependent suppression of the high alcohol intake of chronically intoxicated rats by calcium-acetyl homotaurinate. Alcohol 4: 97–102

Le Magnen J, Tran G, Durlach J (1987b) Lack of effects of calcium-acetyl homotaurinate on chronic and acute toxicities of ethanol in rats. Alcohol 4: 103–108

Lesch OM, Walter H, Fischer F, Platz M, Haring C, Leitner A, Benda N (1994) New developments in reducing alcohol intake. Alcohol Clin Exp Res 18: 43A

Lhuintre JP, Daoust M, Moore ND, Chretien P, Saligaut C, Tran G, Boismare F, Hillemand B (1985) Ability of calcium bis acetyl homotaurine, a GABA agonist, to prevent relapse in weaned alcoholics. Lancet I: 1014–1016

Liljequist S, Borg S (1993) Pharmacotherapy of alcohol and drug dependence. Curr Opin Psychiatr 6/3: 419–423

Littleton JM (1995) Acamprosate; how does it work? Addiction (in press)

Littleton JM, Little HJ (1994) Current concepts of alcohol dependence. Addiction 89: 1397–1412

McCusker CG, Brown K (1995) Cue-exposure to alcohol-associated stimuli reduces autonomic reactivity, but not craving and anxiety in dependent drinkers. Alcohol Alcohol 30: 319–327

Modell JG, Glaser FB, Cyr L, Mountz JM (1992) Obsessive and compulsive characteristics of craving for alcohol in alcohol abuse and dependence. Alcohol Clin Exp Res 16: 272–274

Morgan PF, Nadi NZ, Karamaini J, Linnoila M (1992) Mapping rat brain structures activated during ethanol withdrawal; role of glutamate and NMDA receptors. Eur J Pharmacol M1 225: 217–222

O'Brien CP (1994) Treatment of alcoholism as a chronic disorder. EXS [Exp Suppl] 71: 349–359

O'Brien CP, Childress AR, McLellan T, Ehrman R (1990) Integrating systemic cue exposure with standard treatment in recovering drug dependent patients. Addict Behav 15: 355–365

O'Connor PG, Gottlieb LD, Kraus ML, Segal SR, Horwitz RI (1991) Social and clinical factors as predictors of outcome in outpatient alcohol withdrawal. J Gen Intern Med 6: 312–316

Pelc I, Le Bon O, Verbanck P (1994) Acamprosate in the treatment of alcohol dependence, a six month post-detoxification study. Alcohol Clin Exp Res 18: 38A

Pickens RW, Johanson CE (1992) Craving: consensus of status and agenda for future research. Drug Alcohol Depend 30: 127–131

Poldrugo F, Chabac S, Lehert P (1994) Acamprosate in the long-term treatment of alcoholism: is its use recommended within the psycho-social approach? Alcohol Clin Exp Res 18: 43A

Rassnick S, D'Amico E, Riley E, Pulvirenti L, Ziegelgansberger W, Koob GF (1992) GABA and nucleus accumbens glutamate modulate ethanol self-administration in rats. Ann N Y Acad Sci 654: 502–505

Robbins SJ, Ehrman RN (1992) Designing studies of drug conditioning in humans. Psychopharmacology 106: 143–153

Robinson TE, Berridge KC (1993) The neural basis of craving: an incentive-sensitisation theory of addiction. Brain Res Brain Res Rev 18: 247–291

Rosenhow DJ, Niaura RS, Childress AR, Abrams DB, Monti PM (1990) Cue reactivity in addictive behaviors: theoretical and treatment implications. Int J Addict 25: 957–993

Samson HH, Harris RA (1992) The neurobiology of alcohol abuse. Trends Pharmacol Sci 13: 206–211

Siegel S (1979) The role of conditioning in drug tolerance and addiction. In: (Keehan JD (ed) Psychopathology in animals: research and treatment implications. Academic London, pp 143–168

Steward J, de Wit H, Eikelboom R (1984) The role of un-conditioned and conditioned drug effects in the self-administration of stimulants and opiates. Psychol Rev 91: 251–268

Swift RM, Stout RL (1992) The relationship between craving, anxiety, and other symptoms in opioid withdrawal. J Subst Abuse 4: 19–26

Tran G, Steru L, Daoust M, Parot P, Ladure P, Libert C, Boismare F et al (1990) Acamprosate appears to decrease alcohol intake in weaned alcoholics. Alcohol Alcohol 25: 613–622

Volpicelli JR, Alterman AI, Hayashida M, O'Brien CP (1992) Naltrexone in the treatment of alcohol dependence. Arch Gen Psychiatry 49: 876–880

Wise RA (1988) The neurobiology of craving: implications for the understanding and treatment of addiction. J Abnorm Psychol 97: 118–132

Zeise ML, Kasparow S, Capogna M, Ziegelgansberger W (1990) Calcium diacetylhomotaurinate decreased the action of excitatory amino acids in the rat neocortex in vitro. Prog Clin Biol Res 351: 237–242

Zeise ML, Kasparov S, Capogna M, Ziegelgansberger W (1993) Acamprosate decreases postsynaptic potentials in the rat neocortex: possible involvement of excitatory amino acid receptors. Eur J Pharmacol 231: 47–52

Pharmacodynamics and Pharmacokinetics of Acamprosate: An Overview*

P. Durbin, T. Hulot, and S. Chabac

Chemistry

Acamprosate (calcium acetylaminopropane sulphonate) is the active substance of Campral and has the following chemical structure $(CH_3\text{-}CO\text{-}NH\text{-}CH_2\text{-}CH_2\text{-}CH_2\text{-}SO_3)_2Ca$. The molecular structure is related to biologically active amino acids such as:

- Taurine ($NH_2\text{-}CH_2\text{-}CH_2\text{-}SO_3H$),
- Gamma-aminobutyric acid (GABA), ($NH\text{-}CH_2\text{-}CH_2\text{-}CH_2\text{-}COOH$),
- Glutamic acid $NH_2\text{-}CHCOOH\text{-}CH_2\text{-}CH_2\text{-}COOH$.

The calcium salt confers stability and high hydrophilicity to the molecule and is freely soluble in water and most biological fluids.

Pharmacodynamics

We first describe the general pharmacodynamic effects of acamprosate and its interaction with other compounds acting on the central nervous system (CNS). Its action on alcohol dependence follows, emphasizing experiments related to its mechanism of action.

General Pharmacodynamics

General Effects on the Central Nervous System

Studies of spontaneous motility, exploratory behaviour, and food and water consumption demonstrated that acamprosate did not alter general animal behaviour in the normal situation. A slight hypothermic effect was detected in mice at high doses (220 mg/kg i.p.).

---

*Most data presented in this paper are part of the acamprosate European registration dossier.

Groupe LIPHA, Research and Development Centre, 115 avenue Lacassagne, 69003 Lyon, France

Sedative Effects

A sedative activity was observed in certain stages of chemically induced hyperactivity such as shaking syndrome induced by kainic acid, cerebellar tremors produced by acetylpyridine or harmaline, agitation generated by morphine or amphetamine/chlordiazepoxide combination, and nervous twitches and convulsions induced by gallamine triiodoethylate.

However, acamprosate did not show any sedative or muscle-relaxant activity in naive animals.

Antidepressant Activity

Acamprosate did not exhibit any characteristic antidepressant activity in conventional tests such as the forced swimming test, the tail suspension test, the antagonism of apomorphine-induced righting reflex, stereotypy and hypothermia in the mouse, and the inhibition of reserpine-induced ptosis. However, acamprosate showed some activity in other tests involving interaction with β-adrenergic transmission such as yohimbine toxicity and antagonism of reserpine or oxotremorine-induced hypothermia.

Other CNS Effects

Acamprosate did not show any hypnotic effects in the righting reflex test and did not potentiate barbiturate narcosis in mice when doses of up to 1 g/kg p.o. were administered. It did not show any anti-aggressive effect and was inactive in the four-plate test, which is commonly used to demonstrate benzodiazepine-like anxiolytic activity. It was devoid of any neuroleptic, dopaminergic or anticonvulsant activity. It did not prevent seizures induced by picrotoxine, strychnine or gallamine and did not display anti-petit mal activity by not preventing the cortical hypersynchronisation induced by gamma hydroxybutyrate in rabbits. It did not exhibit any central analgesic activity since it did not increase the reaction time in the hot plate test in mice when administered in doses of up to 400 mg/kg i.p.

General Pharmacodynamics Other Than CNS

The activity of acamprosate on cardiovascular parameters was investigated in several species and models. It had no effect on blood pressure in normotensive rats. A slight reduction in blood pressure was observed in spontaneous hypertensive rats, at doses of 250 mg/kg i.p., but was not confirmed at doses of 1 g/kg per day by oral route over 5 days. The compound had no direct adrenergic-blocking activity since it did not modify the adrenaline effect on cardiovascular parameters.

Peripheral vasodilatation was inhibited by acamprosate in guinea pigs treated with nicotinate. This activity is likely to be due to the calcium part of the molecule, since calcium chloride exerts the same effect. In dogs, it had negligible effects on cardiovascular, respiratory, gastrointestinal or renal parameters at doses up to 100 mg/kg i.v. No anti-inflammatory activity, but slight anti-allergic activity was demonstrated, which might be explained by an antihistamine effect. However, this was not comparable with the action of known antihistamines. No spasmolytic or anticholinergic effects were demonstrated in vitro.

Acamprosate exerts a protective effect on the cell membrane, as demonstrated in rabbit erythrocytes. In vitro, acamprosate prevented the haemolysis of the erythrocyte membranes at a concentration of 1 mmol/l. This was also confirmed in vivo in rats (Beauge et al. 1991; Rinjard et al. 1988).

In conclusion, acamprosate has few central pharmacodynamic effects, and the actions observed in the CNS do not allow categorisation in any known pharmacological class.

Pharmacological Interactions

Potential interactions between acamprosate and drugs likely to be prescribed during and after the alcohol withdrawal period were investigated in rats and mice. No interaction with disulfiram, antidepressants, anxiolytics, neuroleptics, or hypnotics were demonstrated (see Table 1). Interaction studies with disulfiram, diazepam and imipromine have shown no evidence of pharmacodynamic interaction. A 15-day Phase IV study was performed with 591 patients to evaluate the coprescription of acamprosate with other drugs during alcohol withdrawal, especially barbamates, barbiturates, meprobamate, phenobarbitone and oxazepam. No evidence of interaction was demonstrated (Aubin et al. 1995).

Acamprosate and Alcohol Dependence

Chronic consumption of alcohol induces metabolic and neurobiological adaptations intended to oppose the acute effects of alcohol intoxication and restore a functional balance close to physiological requirements. These adaptive modifications represent the state of physiological dependence which becomes pathologically evident when alcohol is withdrawn. It is now agreed that pharmacological intervention can facilitate or even trigger readaptation mechanisms after withdrawal from chronic alcohol consumption. Therefore, such pharmacological interventions could be considered as a therapeutic tool providing assistance to prevent chronic alcoholic patients from relapse.

Animal models have been designed to obtain behaviour mechanisms and neurobiological reaction patterns that are fairly similar to those observed in alcohol-dependent humans. Although these models exclude psychological and cultural factors, they do provide defined conditions to study the effects of a pharmacological compound on biological alcohol dependence.

Table 1. Interaction studies in animals

Drug category	Test	Species	Results
Anticonvulsants			
Phenobarbitone Sodium valproate Diazepam	Pentylenetetrazole-induced convulsions	Mice	No significant interactions up to 400 mg/kg p.o.
Antidepressants			
Imipramine Fluvoxamine	Reserpine ptosis and hypothermia Potentialisation of 5-HTP* effect	Mice	No significant interactions up to 400 mg/kg p.o.
Anxiolytics			
Clorazepate Diazepam Meprobamate Atrium**	Four-plate test	Mice	No significant interactions up to 400 mg/kg p.o.
Neuroleptics			
Haloperidol Sulpiride Tiapride Chlorpromazine	Climbing inhibition test	Mice	No significant interactions up to 400 mg/kg p.o.
Hypnotics			
Butobarbitone	Onset of sleep and sleep duration	Mice	No significant interactions up to 400 mg/kg p.o.
Alcohol-aversive compounds			
Disulfiram	Decrease of blood pressure induced by disulfiram and alcohol combination	Rats	No significant interactions up to 400 mg/kg p.o.

*5-HTP: 5-hydroxytryptophan; **Atrium: febarbamate + difebarbamate + phenobarbitone

Reduction of Voluntary Alcohol Consumption in "Drinker Rats"

Several studies have been conducted in Long Evans rats showing a natural preference for alcohol. After an initial period during which rats had access only to 12% ethanol solution as a drinking fluid, "drinker rats" were selected on the basis of their voluntary alcohol consumption during a 14-day period during which they were given free choice between water and alcohol.

Intraperitoneally or orally administered acamprosate significantly reduced the voluntary alcohol consumption in these rats in a dose-dependent manner after a 10-day latency period (Boismare et al. 1984) (Fig. 1).

Effects of Acamprosate in Alcohol-Dependent Rats

Severe alcohol dependence in rats was achieved by submitting the animals to forced intoxication by gastric ingestion or pulmonary inhalation. In rats made dependent by gastric alcohol intoxication, acamprosate induced a clear and persistent decrease (50%–70%) in their high consumption of alcohol without affecting their water intake (Fig. 2).

Food and drink consumption was not influenced by acamprosate, which

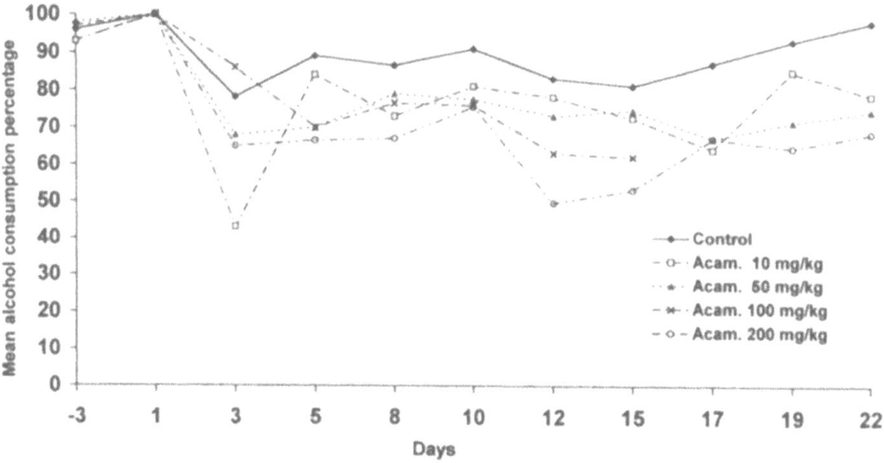

Fig. 1. Voluntary alcohol intake in drinker rats. The figure shows the percentage of alcohol, ingested on each day after the end of treatment with various doses of acamprosate i.p.

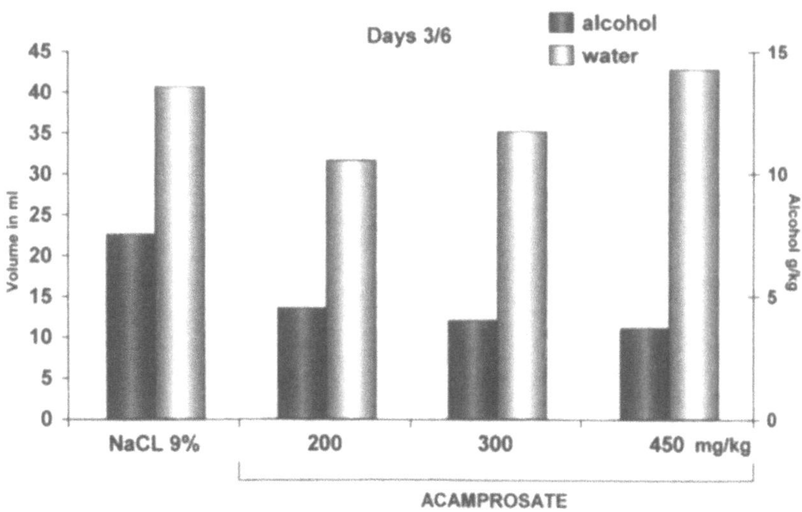

Fig. 2. Effect of acamprosate on alcohol and water consumption

indicated that acamprosate had a specific activity on alcohol intake and not on the satiety feeling, as was reported for serotonin (5HT)-uptake blockers (Gill and Amit 1987). The effect of acamprosate on alcohol consumption was considerably less in alcohol-naive rats than in rats subjected to forced alcohol intake, suggesting that acamprosate interferes with mechanisms leading to alcohol dependence (Le Magnen et al. 1987b).

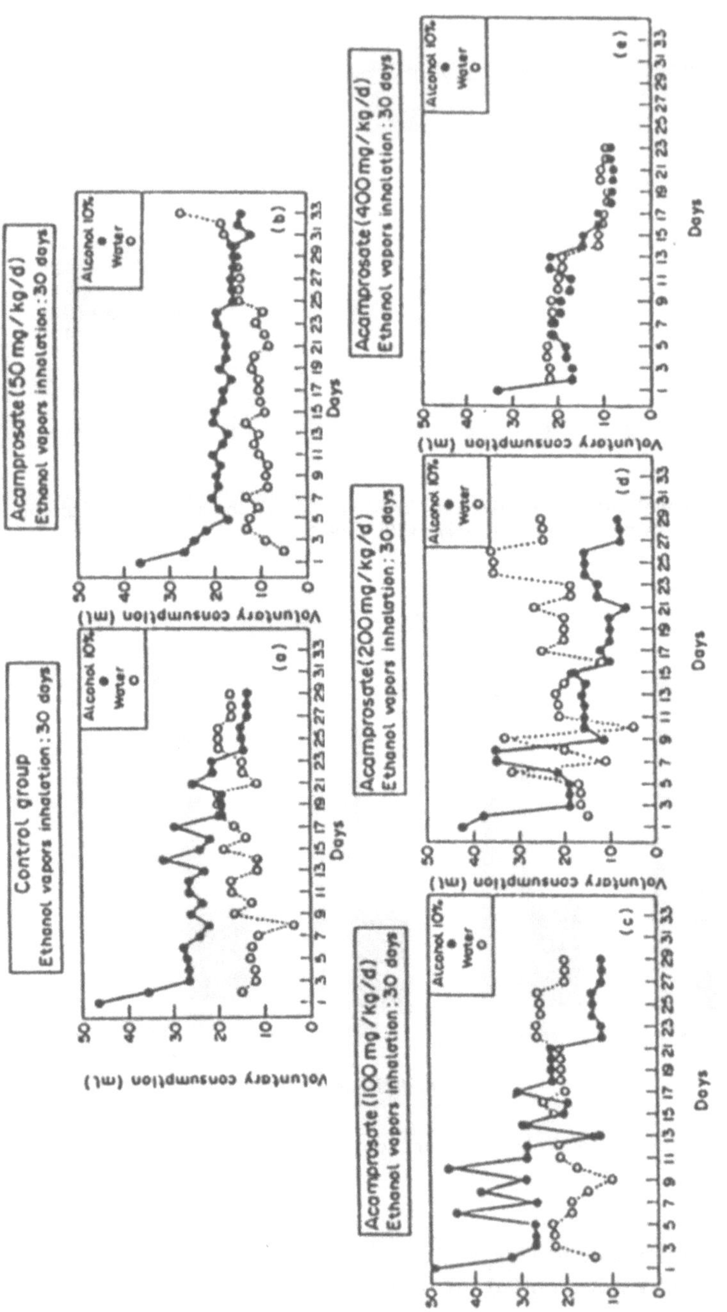

Fig. 3. Alcohol and water consumptions of alcoholised untreated rats (control group) (a) and rats treated with acamprosate 50 mg/kg/d (b), 100 mg/kg/d (c), 200 mg/kg/d (d) and 400 mg/kg/d (e) as expressed in a free-choice beverage procedure

In the pulmonary inhalation model, rats were placed in an alcohol exposure chamber where the atmosphere contained a fixed concentration of ethanol. After this induction period, the rats were given a free choice between pure water and a 10% or 15% alcohol solution as drinking fluid. Voluntary alcohol consumption was measured in control rats and in animals treated with oral acamprosate. Acamprosate selectively reduced alcohol intake in a dose-dependent manner (Fig. 3); a dose of 400 mg/kg completely suppressed alcohol intake (Gewiss et al. 1991).

Acamprosate not only decreased alcohol consumption in a dose-dependent way but also decreased the duration of alcohol overconsumption, i.e. the period when rats consumed more alcohol than water. Lag time to reduce alcohol preference was 23 days, 13 days, and 11 days with 50, 100, and 200 mg/kg acamprosate, respectively. Acamprosate 400 mg/kg immediately suppressed preference for alcohol (Fig. 4).

Effects of Acamprosate on Alcohol Withdrawal

Since at the central level, acamprosate exhibits a protective effect in animals showing hyperactivity (see "Sedative Effects" above), these sedative-like properties could be of interest in reducing some of the physiological manifestations of alcohol withdrawal. This hypothesis has been investigated in alcoholized C57BL mice in which acamprosate at doses of up to 100 mg/kg attenuated convulsions caused by alcohol withdrawal (Gutierrez et al. 1987). Further studies have confirmed this activity (Littleton et al. 1988).

If given during the alcoholization period, acamprosate was also shown to suppress the hyperactivity induced by alcohol withdrawal. This confirmed once more that acamprosate interferes with the mechanisms underlying the development of alcohol dependence (Gewiss et al. 1991).

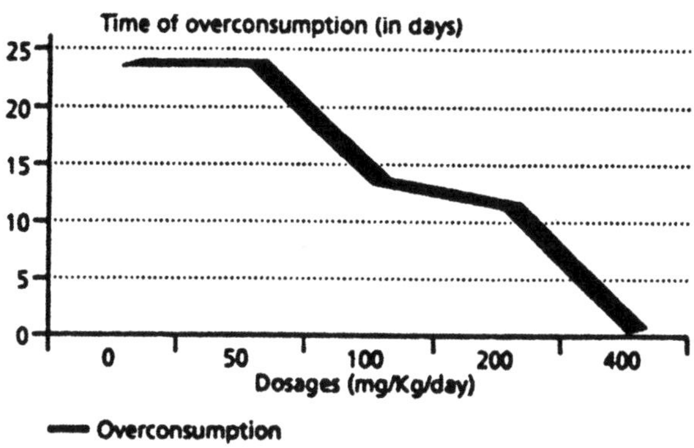

Fig. 4. Drug-dependent time of overconsumption in untreated rats (control group) and rats treated with various doses of acamprosate

Mechanism of Action

Alcohol Toxicity

A possible explanation for the observed reduction in alcohol consumption by acamprosate could be that it potentiates alcohol toxicity. Therefore, the action of acamprosate on the toxic effect of alcohol and its major metabolite acetaldehyde was investigated in a series of specific studies in rodents. Acamprosate did not reveal any reinforcement of the effects of acute alcohol toxicity as expressed by hypothermia and by alcohol-induced motor disturbances (Le Magnen et al. 1987a; Durlach et al. 1988).

Disulfiram or cyanamide exert their alcohol-aversive effects by inhibiting aldehyde dehydrogenase activity which leads to an enhancement of acetaldehyde side effects. Compared with these two compounds, acamprosate does not modify the activity of hepatic aldehyde dehydrogenase in rats at doses up to 400 mg/kg p.o. (Fig. 5). Moreover, acamprosate has been shown to protect mice from the hypomotility induced by high intravenous does of acetaldehyde. From these results, it can be concluded that the reduction of alcohol consumption induced by acamprosate is not due to aversive reactions induced by increasing ethanol or acetaldehyde toxicity in the animal (Durlach et al. 1988).

Activity on the GABAergic System

The role of GABAergic transmission in alcohol drinking and dependence has received much attention. It is commonly agreed that ethanol stimulates the inhibitory effect of GABAergic transmission mainly by acting on $GABA_A$ receptors. If alcohol exposure becomes chronic, adaptive mechanisms are triggered, leading to a reduction in GABAergic transmission (Korpi 1994).

Administration of the GABA antagonist bicucullin concomitantly with acamprosate blocked its effect on voluntary alcohol intake (Boismare et al. 1984). This pioneer observation prompted the early hypothesis that acamprosate shows a GABAergic activity. Further studies demonstrated that acamprosate does possess a GABAergic-like effect. In rats, acamprosate reduced cyclic GMP levels in the cerebellum (Daoust et al. 1985), increased the number of sites for GABA uptake, and modified the affinity of the transporter and GABA uptake rate (Daoust et al. 1984, 1990). Moreover, acamprosate prolonged the survival time of animals given a lethal dose of pentetrazole or bicucullin. Finally, in an in vivo study, acamprosate administered p.o. to alcoholized rats, modified brain GABA transmission (Daoust et al. 1992).

However, although this GABAergic effect was confirmed in humans (Gerra et al. 1992), it is not comparable to that of barbiturates or benzodiazepines. It appears unlikely that GABAergic properties of acamprosate could explain its effect on alcohol dependence. According to the general pharmacodynamic observations, acamprosate is far from being a GABA agonist like the benzodiazepines or barbiturates are. Moreover, acamprosate cannot be a substitute for GABA agonists in a drug-discrimination procedure (Grant and Woolverton

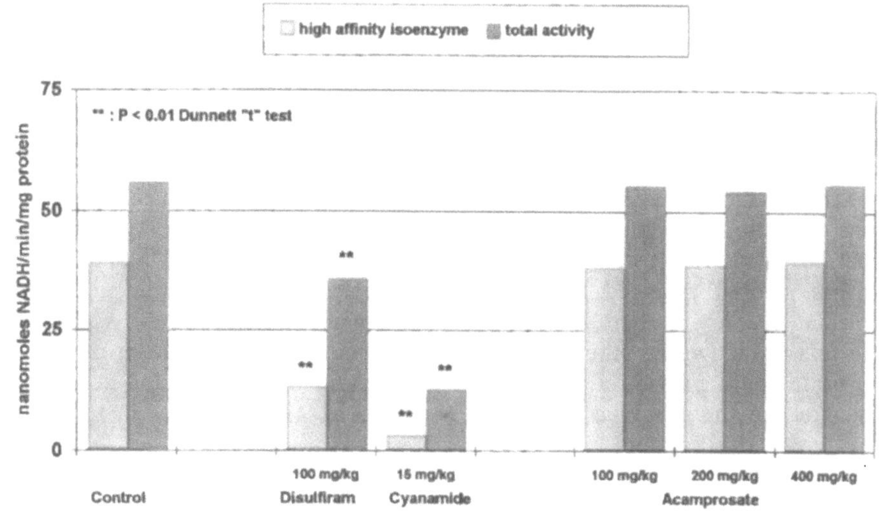

Fig. 5a,b. Compared effect of acamprosate, disulfiram and cyanamide on rat hepatic aldehyde dehydrogenase activity. **a** Total activity. **b** High-affinity isoenzyme activity

1989). The GABAergic-like properties of acamprosate are likely to contribute to its action on alcohol dependence, but other effect(s) would probably take place upstream.

Activity on Excitatory Amino-Acids

A body of evidence shows that excitatory amino-acids of the glutamate type are also involved in alcohol dependence. Together with a reduction of the inhibitory effect of GABA, chronic ethanol intake induces an increase in excitatory transmission, mainly through *N*-methyl-D-aspartic acid (NMDA) receptors which become more functional and counterbalance the GABA hypoexcitability (Samson and Harris 1992; Tsai et al. 1995). Moreover NMDA receptor antagonists have been shown to reduce ethanol self-administration in rats (Rassnick et al. 1992).

Therefore, encouraged by the chemical similarity of acamprosate with glutamate or homocysteate, investigators studied the effects of acamprosate on excitatory amino-acids transmission in several models. In 1990, Zeise et al. showed in vitro that acamprosate reduced post-synaptic potentials and the depolarizing response evoked by iontophoretic application of several excitatory amino-acid receptor agonists (Zeise et al. 1990, 1993). Cultured bovine adrenal cells release catecholamines following stimulation by various excitatory amino acids, predominantly by acting on NMDA receptors. When added to bovine adrenal cells 30 min before NMDA or homocysteic acid, acamprosate caused a dramatic inhibition of catecholamine release (Bouchenafa et al. 1990).

Further studies showed that without directly binding to NMDA receptors, acamprosate could reduce the hyperexcitatory activity of the amino-acids of the glutamate type observed at the interruption of alcohol intake. In vitro, acamprosate increases synaptosomal ^{3}H-glutamate uptake in rat hippocampus and striatum. This effect was confirmed in vivo in normal and alcoholised rats (Daoust et al. 1991).

Beyond the fact that the excitatory amino-acid antagonism closely fits the pharmacodynamic properties of acamprosate, such a mechanism could explain the reduction in hyperexcitability which occurs during the post-withdrawal period. Moreover, it was suggested that "craving", i.e. the irresistible desire to drink alcohol reported by alcoholic patients after withdrawal, would be mediated, at least in part, by excitatory amino-acids (Littleton 1995). According to this attractive hypothesis, the excitatory amino-acid antagonism of acamprosate could provide a biochemical explanation of the reducing action on alcohol craving observed in humans (Lesch et al. 1994; Paille et al. 1995; see M. Soyka, this volume).

Other Transmitters, Other Targets

Acamprosate failed to show significant effects on other neurotransmitter systems like dopamine or acetylcholine. Several studies investigated the effect of acamprosate on 5HT transmission, but the modifications observed were often contradictory (Daoust et al. 1989; Rouhani et al. 1988; Durlach 1987), thus suggesting that 5HT would not play a key role in acamprosate action. It was also pointed out that the way acamprosate interferes with membranes might lie behind its effect on neurotransmission (Rinjard et al. 1988; Beauge et al. 1991). However, such a mechanism would suffer from a lack of specificity.

One interesting method of investigation is to look for the drug action site. Acamprosate appears to be present in all areas of the rat brain after crossing the blood-brain barrier (Durbin and Belleville 1995), and there are also reports that it binds on specific sites in the hippocampus (Daoust et al. 1993). There is no doubt in the near future, the characterisation of this/these site(s) will offer new opportunities to define acamprosate's mechanism of action more precisely. Recently, acamprosate has been reported to increase taurine release in the rat brain in vivo (Dahchour et al. 1994) and to interfere with calcium-channel protein (Al Qatari and Littleton 1995). These two observations may offer further promising insights since they could be related to hyperexcitability, taurine being an inhibitory amino acid, and calcium the intracellular mediator of neuronal excitation.

In conclusion, whatever the transmission systems involved, the seemingly various actions of acamprosate in the brain appear to point towards neuronal excitability. Thus, up to now, acamprosate can be considered as a stabilising agent that removes the bursts of hyperexcitability which frequently occur in abstinent alcoholic patients and thereby preventing them from relapse.

Pharmacokinetics

The main pharmacokinetic characteristics of acamprosate were investigated in studies with several animal models and in humans.

Animal Pharmacokinetics

Studies were performed in rats, rabbits and dogs following single oral and intravenous administration, and in mice, rats and dogs following repeated oral administration. Labelled and unlabelled acamprosate were used in these studies to define the drug's main pharmacokinetic parameters.

Absorption and Plasma Kinetics

From these studies, it was confirmed that acamprosate is rapidly absorbed through the gastrointestinal tract, although to a limited extent. Slight differences in the absorption and bioavailability of acamprosate were found in rat, dog and rabbit models.

After oral administration, acamprosate rapidly appears in plasma, and its levels are detectable for up to 30 h. Acamprosate can be detected in plasma 15–30 min after oral administration to rats and dogs. The bioavailability of acamprosate after oral administration does not exceed 16% in rats. In dogs, the bioavailability after oral administration of acamprosate at the dose of 25 mg/kg is 60%.

Distribution

It was shown that acamprosate is widely distributed throughout the tissues in rats and dogs, although low concentrations are found in individual tissues.

After administration of ^{14}C acamprosate, the radioactivity levels in the liver and the kidney exceeded those found in plasma, while in other tissues the radioactivity level was inferior to those found in plasma. Ninety-six hours after administration, radioactivity was not detectable.

It was also observed that acamprosate is able to cross the placental barrier during the period of organogenesis and can be found in the milk of lactating rats. Acamprosate also crosses the rat blood-brain barrier and is found in all brain areas (Durbin and Belleville 1995).

Metabolism

Samples of pooled urine and faeces from rats, dogs and rabbits were analysed using high-performance liquid chromatography (HPLC) after single oral administration of labelled acamprosate to determine whether or not acamprosate is metabolised. The results showed only a single radiocomponent identical to acamprosate in both urine and faeces. These findings thus suggest that acamprosate is not metabolised.

Excretion

It was found that acamprosate is eliminated from the plasma by the kidneys within the first 120 h after oral administration. Seventy-two hours after intravenous administration of acamprosate to rats, 90% of the administered dose is found in the urine and 8.6% in the faeces. The probable mechanism of excretion is by glomerular filtration. The presence of acamprosate in the faeces after oral administration can be attributed to unabsorbed acamprosate, but, biliary and/or intestinal secretion may also occur.

Human Pharmacokinetics

The pharmacokinetics of acamprosate in humans were investigated in young healthy adult male volunteers after oral and intravenous administration at various dosages. The influence of acamprosate on the kinetics of ethyl alcohol, and the effect of ethanol upon the pharmacokinetics of acamprosate were also evaluated. In addition, the pharmacokinetics of acamprosate in alcoholic patients who had completed alcohol-withdrawal treatment were assessed, as were the influence of food and effect of gender on acamprosate pharmacokinetics after single oral administration and the kinetics of acamprosate in patients with liver disease and chronic renal failure. Finally, interaction studies with psychotropic drugs (benzodiazepines, antidepressants, neuroleptics and disulfiram) were performed.

Analysis

Apart from two studies with radiolabelled acamprosate and two studies in which an HPLC assay was used, a standard assay method with gas chromatography-mass spectrometry (GC/MS) and with negative chemical ionisation was used for determining acetylhomotaurine is plasma and urine. The lower limit of detection for acetylhomotaurine is 5 ng/ml.

Absorption and Plasma Kinetics

In healthy males, acamprosate tablets are partly absorbed through the gastrointestinal tract but there is an important interindividual variation. The lengthy absorption time indicates a slow and prolonged absorption through the intestinal tract. There is a linear relationship between the dose, C_{max} and

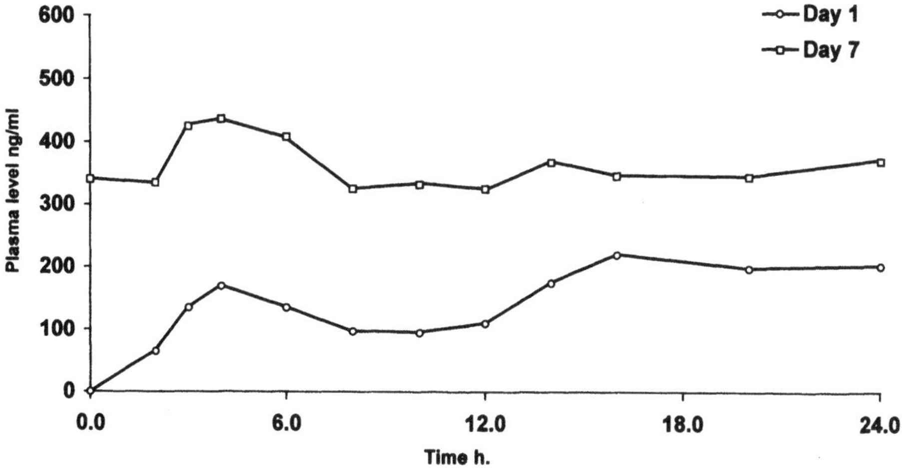

Fig. 6. Plasma concentrations of acamprosate on day 1 and day 7 of administration of 2 × 333 mg three times daily in healthy volunteers

$AUC_{0-\infty}$. Steady state levels of acethylhomotaurine are achieved by the 7th day of dosing (Fig. 6).

There is no significant difference in the plasma pharmacokinetics of acamprosate between male and female subjects.

Distribution and Metabolism

It must be pointed out that acamprosate does not bind to plasma proteins. In a study conducted with ^{14}C acamprosate, the HPLC analysis of faecal and urine samples showed that acamprosate does not appear to be metabolised. These results are in accordance with those obtained in animals.

Excretion and Elimination

Ninety percent of an intravenously administered dose of acamprosate is eliminated in the urine by glomerular filtration within 24 h. After oral and intravenous dosing, the apparent half-life values are 13.0 h and 3.2 h, respectively, underlying a flip-flop absorption process which is consistent with prolonged absorption.

Pharmacokinetics in Patients

The pharmacokinetic parameters for weaned alcoholoc patients were also evaluated for validation purposes. Serial plasma levels of acamprosate were

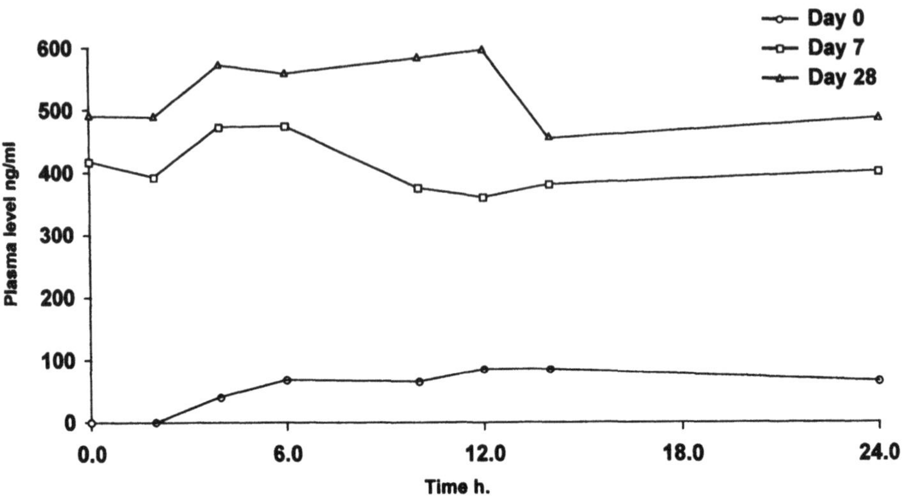

Fig. 7. Mean plasma concentrations of acamprosate on day 1, day 7 and day 28 in patients treated with acamprosate 2 × 333 mg tablets three times daily

determined on the 1st, 7th and 28th day of dosing with acamprosate 1998 mg/day in patients who had completed alcohol withdrawal therapy. After one week of treatment acamprosate values in plasma in weaned alcoholics were found to be very similar to those observed in volunteers. In addition, a further increase in plasma levels of acamprosate at day 28 in comparison to those obtained at day 7 was detected. Therefore, it can be concluded that the kinetics of acamprosate in alcohol-dependent patients who had completed withdrawal therapy are similar to those observed in healthy adult volunteers (Fig. 7).

Interactions with Food and Ethanol

When acamprosate is given orally as a single dose in non-fasting conditions, its bioavailability is decreased by 20% as shown by C_{max} and AUC values (Fig. 8).

It should be noted that in all clinical studies, acamprosate tablets were administered three times daily with food. It is unlikely that food will influence plasma concentrations of acetylhomotaurine once steady state levels are achieved.

Two studies were completed which demonstrated that administering acamprosate tablets 666 mg t.i.d. for 2 days did not influence the pharmacokinetic parameters of ethanol when 80 ml of 40% whisky were ingested 2 h after the final dose of acamprosate. Similarly, the pharmacokinetic parameters of acetylhomotaurine were not influenced by a concomitant ingestion of alcohol (Fig. 9).

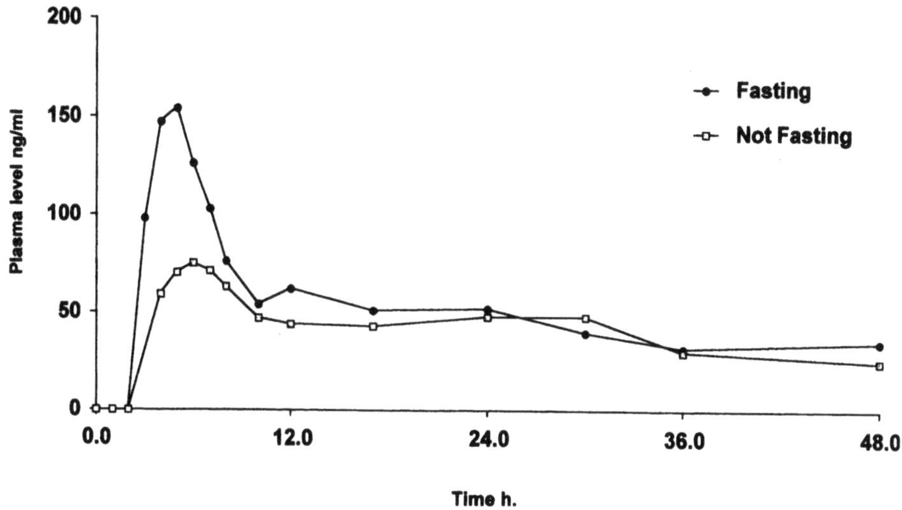

Fig. 8. Mean acamprosate plasma concentrations after a single oral administration of acamprosate in fasting and nonfasting subjects

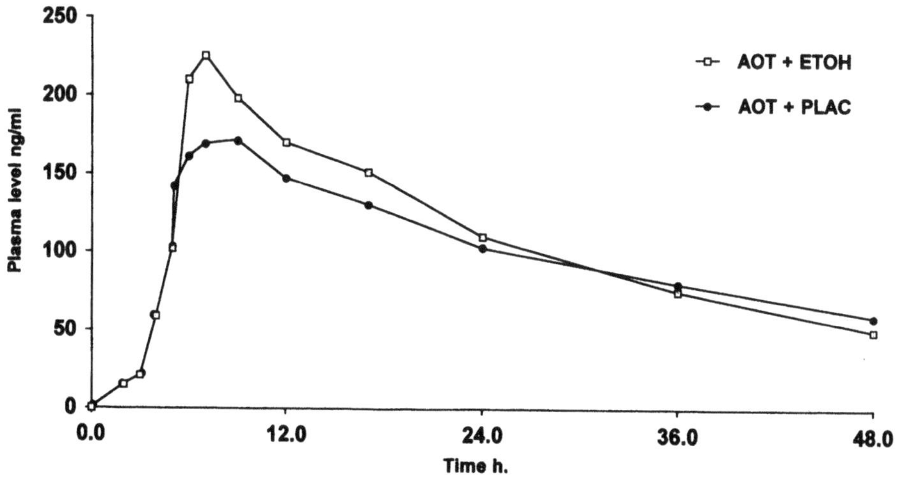

Fig. 9. Plasma concentrations of acamprosate after oral administration of a single acamprosate dose with or without ethanol

Pharmacokinetics in Hepatic or Renal Dysfunction

The pharmacokinetic parameters of acamprosate are not modified by hepatic dysfunction, as confirmed in patients at different stages of alcohol-induced liver insufficiency.

In line with probable acetylhomotaurine excretion through the kidney, studies have confirmed a linear relationship between creatinine clearance and total apparent plasma clearance, renal clearance, plasma half-life and the mean residence time of acetylhomotaurine. Consequently, acamprosate is contraindicated in patients with renal dysfunction.

Interaction with Other Drugs

Potential interactions between acamprosate and drugs likely to be prescribed for and during the maintenance of alcohol deprivation were investigated in humans. Results showed a lack of pharmacokinetic interaction with diazepam, imipramine and disulfiram. The concomitant administration of disulfiram and benzodiazepines, antidepressants and other psychotropic drugs with acamprosate has also frequently occurred in the clinical trials performed in phases II, III, and IV. In all these studies, there has been no evidence of any pharmacological or clinical drug interaction.

Conclusion

Several animal experimental studies have demonstrated that acamprosate decreases ethanol consumption in several "alcoholism" models using either alcohol-dependent or preferring rats.

The similarity of the acamprosate chemical structure with endogenous amino acid neurotransmitters endows the compound with great potential to interfere in neurotransmission. Acamprosate was shown to exhibit GABAergic activity and to antagonize excitatory amino acid transmission.

Chronic alcohol absorption trigggers neuroadaptative modifications to help maintain a physiological function. Acting on both excitatory and inhibitory systems, acamprosate helps the CNS to restore excitation/inhibition equilibrium that is lost after cessation of alcohol absorption.

Although the targets on which acamprosate acts are not yet fully identified at the molecular level, several pieces of the puzzle are already known. They all appear to be related to the regulation of neuronal hyperexcitability. Further studies are ongoing which should soon help to identify the mechanism of action.

Acamprosate's pharmacokinetic profile in humans is characterized by limited but sustained absorption. After oral administration, steady state is reached rapidly (1 week). The compound is neither bound to plasma proteins nor metabolized, and it is excreted in urine. In patients, the kinetic profile is identical to that of healthy volunteers. It is neither modified by alcohol intake nor by hepatic dysfunction. There is no kinetic interaction between acamprosate and the various other types of treatment likely to be prescribed simultaneously (e.g.) (diazepam, imipramine, and disulfiram).

Acamprosate is a promising therapy in treatment of alcoholism. It represents not only a hope for chronic alcoholic patients, but is also a new tool to improve our knowledge of alcohol dependence.

References

Al-Qatari M, Littleton J (1995) The anti-craving drug acamprosate inhibits calcium channel antagonist binding to membranes from rat cerebral cortex. Alcohol Alcohol 30(4): 551

Aubin HJ, Lehert P, Beaupere B, Parot P, Barrucand D (1995) Tolerability of the combination of acamprosate with drugs used to prevent alcohol withdrawal syndrome. Alcoholism 31(1-2): 25-38

Beauge F, Achard S, Niel E, Durbin P (1991) Acamprosate interactions with ethanol effects on biological membranes. A preliminary fluorescence polarization study. Alcohol Alcohol 26(2): 235

Boismare F, Daoust M, Moore ND, Saligaut C, Lhuintre JP, Chretien P, Durlach JA (1984) Homotaurine derivative reduces the voluntary intake of ethanol by rats: are cerebral GABA receptors involved?. Pharmacol Biochem Behav 21(5): 787-789

Bouchenafa O, Cwynarski K, Littleton J (1990) Interactions between excitatory amino acids and aotal in a cell culture model of ethanol dependence. Alcohol Clin Exp Res 14(2): 312

Dahchour A, Quertemont E, Durbin P, De Witte P (1994) Acute ethanol increases taurine in the nucleus accumbens but not glutamate nor GABA = Microdialysis study. 7th ESBRA Congress, Queensland, Australia, 26 June-1 July, 1994; 33A-no 5.14

Daoust M, Saligaut C, Moore ND, Chretien P, Boismare F (1984) Effet de l'acétyl homotaurinate de calcium sur les constantes des cinétiques d'accumulation de 3H GABA dans les synaptosomes striataux de rats préférant l'alcool. J Pharmacol 15(4): 458-459

Daoust M, Lhuintre JP, Saligaut C, Chretien P, Moore ND, Boismare F (1985) Calcium bis acétyl homotaurine (Ca AOTA):un nouvel agoniste gabaergique? J Pharmacol 16(4): 521

Daoust M, Protais P, Boucly P, Tran G, Rinjard P, Dokhan R, Fillion G (1989) Intervention of AOTAL on serotoninergic and noradrenergic system. Alcohol Alcohol 24(4): 370

Daoust M, Legrand E, Tran G, Durbin P, Gewiss M, Heidbreder C, De Witte P (1990) Acamprosate treatment differentially modulates synaptosomal gaba uptake in chronically alcoholized rats. Alcohol Clin Exp Res 14(2): 281

Daoust M, Legrand E, Aubin N, Durbin P (1991) Acamprosate increases, in vitro, 3H-glutamate synaptosomal uptake without affecting glutamate release. Alcohol Alcohol 26(2): 239

Daoust M, Legrand E, Gewiss M, Heidbreder C, De Witte P, Tran G, Durbin P (1992) Acamprosate modulates synaptosomal GABA transmission in chronicallly alcoholised rats. Pharmacol Biochem Behav 41(4): 669-674

Daoust M, Legrand E, Durbin P (1993) 3H-Acamprosate (AOTAL) binding in hippocampal membrane preparation of alcoholism rats. Alcohol Alcohol 28(2): C2.9

Durbin P, Belleville M (1995) Rat pharmacokinetic profile of acamprosate in plasma, brain and CSF. Alcohol Alcohol 30(4): 548

Durlach J (1987) Le N acétyl homotaurinate de calcium: une thérapeutique nouvelle de l'alcoolisme à sites d'action pharmacologique multiple. French-Italian joint meeting on medical chemistry, Pisa, Italy, 22-26 Sept, 1987

Durlach J, Rinjard P, Sprince H, Smith G (1988) Similar antagonist effects of Ca N-acetylhomotaurinate on depression of motor activity and lethality induced by acetaldehyde or ethanol. Methods Find Exp Clin Pharmacol 10(7): 437-447

Gerra G, Caccavari R, Delsignore R, Vourna S, Maestra D, Ugolotti G, Passeri M (1992) Pituitary responses to CA-acetyl homotaurinate in normal subjects and alcoholics. Neuroendocrinol Lett 14(2): 119-126

Gewiss M, Heidbreder C, Opsomer L, Durbin P, De Witte P (1991) Acamprosate and diazepam differentially modulate alcohol-induced behavioural and cortical alterations in rats following chronic inhalation of ethanol vapour. Alcohol Alcohol 26(2): 129-137

Gill K, Amit Z (1987) Effects of serotonin uptake blockade on food water and ethanol consumption in rats. Alcohol Clin Exp Res 11(5): 444-449

Grant KA, Woolverton WL (1989) Reinforcing and discriminative stimulus effects of Ca-acetyl homotaurine in animals. Pharmacol Biochem Behav 32(3): 607-611

Gutierrez S, Daoust M, Rinjard P, Lhuintre JP, Boismare F (1987) L'acétylhomotaurinate de calcium, molécule à propriétés gabaergiques, atténue le syndrome de sevrage alcoolique chez la souris C57BL. Rev Alcool 32(4): 241-247

Korpi ER (1994) Role of $GABA_A$ receptors in the actions of alcohol and in alcoholism : recent advances. Alcohol Alcohol 29(2): 115-129

Le Magnen J, Tran G, Durlach J (1987a) Lack of effects of Ca-acetyl homotaurinate on chronic and acute toxicities of ethanol in rats. Alcohol 4(2): 103-108

Le Magnen J, Tran G, Durlach J, Martin C (1987b) Dose-dependent suppression of the high alcohol intake of chronically intoxicated rats by Ca-acetyl homotaurinate. Alcohol 4(2): 97–102

Lesch OM, Walter W, Fischer P, Platz W, Haring C, Leitner A, Benda N (1994) Acamprosate helps to reduce craving. Annual Scientific Meeting of the research society on alcoholism, RSA, Maui, Hawaii, 18–23 June, 1994, 464–no. 265

Littleton J (1995) Acamprosate in alcohol dependence: how does it work. Addiction 90: 1179–1188

Littleton JM, Dunnage J, Pagonis C (1988) Alcohol dependence and modulation of neuronal calcium channels. In: Kuriyama K, Takada A, Ishu H (eds) Biomedical and Social Aspects of Alcohol and Alcoholism Elsevier, Amsterdam, pp 229–234

Paille F, Guelfi JD, Perkins A, Royer RJ, Steru L, Parot P (1995) Double-blind randomized multicentre trial of acamprosate in maintaining abstinence from alcohol. Alcohol Alcohol 30(2): 239–247

Rassnick S, Damico E, Riley E, Pulvirenti L, Zeglgansberger W, Koob GF (1992) GABA and nucleus accumbens glutamate neurotransmission modulate ethanol self-administration in rats. Ann New York Acad Sci 654: 502–505

Rinjard P, Alcindor LG, Ladure P, Durlach P, Tran G (1988) Effects of withdrawal on the C/P molar ratio and phospholipase activities in erythrocyte membranes of AOTA-Ca treated ethanol fed rats. Alcohol Alcohol 23(3): A35

Rouhani S, Tran G, Durlach J, Leplaideur F, Emmanouilidis E, Poenaru S (1988) Vigilance states (VS) and cerebral monoaminergic (CMA) metabolism in the alcohol treated rat (RETOH): effect of calcium acetyl homotaurinate (Ca-AOTA). In: Kuriyama K, Takada A, Ishu H (eds) Biomedical and Social Aspects of Alcohol and Alcoholism. Elsevier, Amsterdam, pp 243–246

Samson HH, Harris RA (1992) The neurobiology of alcohol abuse. TIPS 13: 206–211

Tsai G, Gastfriend DR, Coyle JT (1995) The glutamaergic basis of human alcoholism. AMJ Psychiatr 152(3): 332–340

Zeise ML, Kasparow S, Capogna M, Zieglgansberger W (1990) Calciumdiacetylhomotaurinate (Ca-AOTA) decreases the action of excitatory amino acids in the rat neocortex in vitro. Prog Clin Biol Res 351: 237–242

Zeise ML, Kasparov S, Capogna M, Zieglgansberger W (1993) Acamprosate (calciumacetylhomotaurinate) decreases postsynaptic potentials in the rat neocortex: possible involvement of excitatory amino acid receptors. Eur J Pharmacol 231(1): 47–52

Actions of Acamprosate on Neurons of the Central Nervous System

W. Zieglgänsberger[1], C. Hauser[1], C. Wetzel[1], J. Putzke[1], G.R. Siggins[2], and R. Spanagel[1]

Introduction

The mechanism behind the intoxicating and the addictive properties of ethanol most likely derives from distinct cellular mechanisms. In recent years the emphasis has shifted from the hypothesis that alcohol disorganizes or "fluidizes" membranes to voltage-gated ion channels or channels gated by neurotransmitters. Cholinergic and serotonergic mechanisms are affected by alcohol administration at concentrations which also inhibit the action of excitatory amino acid transmitters (EAA) such as L-glutamate, enhance GABAergic synaptic transmission at various sites in the central nervous system through an action on $GABA_A$ receptors, or inhibit voltage-sensitive Ca^{2+} channels. Chronic alcohol treatment increases the density of *N*-methyl-D-aspartate (NMDA) receptors (e.g., Sanna et al. 1993) and voltage-sensitive Ca^{2+} channels (Guppy and Littleton 1994) in central neurons whereas $GABA_A$ receptor mediated actions are reduced (Samson and Harris 1992). These changes provide a plausible explanation for the hyperactivity resulting from alcohol withdrawal.

The cellular study of drugs known to be effective in reducing alcoholism, such as acamprosate (calcium acetyl-homotaurinate; Lipha, France), may lead in the direction of a better understanding of alcohol dependence and to further refinement of anticraving agents (Zeise et al. 1990, 1993; Zieglgänsberger and Zeise 1992). Clinical studies have already shown that acamprosate is very successful in preventing relapse in weaned alcoholics (Lhuintre et al. 1985, 1990; Ladewig et al. 1993).

Current research suggests that ethanol-induced long-term changes in the excitability of central neurons involve the activation of the genome. The activity-dependent modulation of gene expression by immediate-early genes (IEGs) is a characteristic feature of highly integrated systems and greatly expands the capacity to react in a more plastic manner to environmental stimuli. This stimulus transcription coupling is probably the basis for long-term responses of neurons which contribute to such phenomena as regeneration, learning, neuronal plasticity, and persisting drug effects. Acamprosate clearly

[1]Max-Planck-Institut für Psychiatrie, Klinisches Institut, Kraepelinstr. 2, 80804 München, Germany
[2]The Scripps Research Institute, Department of Neuropharmacology, 10666 North Torrey Pines Road, La Jolla, CA 92037, USA

affects IEG expression and the expression of genes coding for EAA receptor subunits in various brain regions of the rat.

Acamprosate and Excitatory Amino Acid Transmitters

L-Glutamate fulfills all criteria for classification as a major excitatory neurotransmitter in the central nervous system (CNS); probably only a few neurons in the CNS do not receive EAA-mediated synaptic input. Glutamatergic synaptic transmission involves the activation of ionotropic and metabotropic receptor subtypes. By far the most fully characterized L-glutamate receptor subtype is the NMDA receptor (Westbrook 1994; Hollmann and Heinemann 1994).

When acamprosate was perfused in therapeutically relevant concentrations to an in vitro slice preparation of the rat neocortex, it reduced excitatory and inhibitory postsynaptic potentials and the depolarizing responses evoked by iontophoretic application of the EAAs, L-glutamate, L-aspartate, L-homocysteate, and NMDA (Zeise et al. 1993). Acamprosate decreased electrical excitability of neocortical neurons without apparently changing their membrane potential, input resistance, after-hyperpolarization, or threshold and amplitude of the action potential. In vivo iontophoretic and systemic administration of acamprosate reduced the extracellularly recorded unit activity elicited by iontophoretically applied EAAs, whereas spontaneous discharges remained unaffected. In hippocampal CA1 pyramidal neurons (Madamba et al. 1995) and nucleus accumbens neurons (Berton et al. 1995), where acamprosate also did not affect membrane potential or input resistance, it significantly increased the NMDA component of excitatory postsynaptic potentials and increased inward current responses in some CA1 neurons to exogenous NMDA. A synopsis of these data suggests that this compound may act postsynaptically to increase the NMDA component of excitatory transmission in hippocampal CA1 pyramidal neurons. In this area (Siggins et al. 1987), as in the nucleus accumbens (Nie et al. 1993, 1994), which is a structure thought to play a major role in drug reinforcement, ethanol reduces excitatory and inhibitory postsynaptic potentials. In contrast to acamprosate, ethanol also potently decreases NMDA-induced currents in CA1 hippocampal CA1 pyramidal neurons (Lovinger et al. 1989) and nucleus accumbens neurons (Nie et al. 1994).

Acamprosate and GABA

Recent evidence has cast some doubt on the GABA-activated chloride channel as a primary locus of action of ethanol (Kalant 1993; Littleton and Little 1994). The question of whether GABA interactions play a direct role in ethanol intoxication is still unanswered, because to date very few studies have revealed an ethanol effect on endogenous, synaptically released GABA. Until now most studies have been concerned primarily with GABA acting at the $GABA_A$ receptor. However, the role of $GABA_B$ receptors in alcohol intoxication or alcoholism is also coming into discussion (e.g., Proctor and Dunwiddie 1991;

Proctor et al. 1992). Alcohol enhances the inhibitory actions of GABA mediated through the $GABA_A$ receptor in various, but not all, central neurons (Soldo et al. 1994). One reason for these findings might be an alternative subunit composition of the GABA receptor in different regions. In some preparations acamprosate modifies or mimics GABAergic (Boismare et al. 1984a,b, 1986; Gewiss et al. 1991; Daoust et al. 1992) or opioidergic mechanisms (Le Magnen et al. 1987). In rat neocortical neurons in vitro and transfected human embryonic kidney cells (HEK 293) acamprosate did not alter the responses to γ-aminobutyric acid. The cells were recorded in the whole-cell voltage-clamp configuration using the giga-seal technique, and the compounds were locally applied via a multibarrel/single-tip superfusion device. Acamprosate affected neither the peak amplitude nor the time constant of desensitization of the GABA-induced currents in $\alpha_1\beta_2\gamma_2$ or in $\alpha_6\beta_2\gamma_2$ subunit containing $GABA_A$ receptors. Acamprosate did not bind to $GABA_A$ receptors (containing either the α_1 or the α_6-$GABA_A$ receptor subunit) or to glycine receptors in these cells and does not, in contrast to flunitrazepam, enhance Cl^- currents (in α_1-containing receptors). These data clearly indicate that acamprosate has no "benzodiazepine-like" potential in these cells (Zieglgänsberger et al. 1995).

Acamprosate and the Expression of IEGs and EAA Receptor Subunits

Transcriptional modulators encoded by IEGs are induced as a response to short-term receptor activation or to changes in membrane potential and probably form the basis for long-term responses including persisting drug effects. The IEGs carry regulatory sequences necessary for induction through second messenger systems (Hunt et al. 1995).

Acamprosate reduces the expression of the *c-fos* gene coding for transcriptional modulators in withdrawal and postwithdrawal periods (Putzke et al. 1996). It is feasible to assume that through such actions acamprosate could counteract the long-lasting changes in latent neuronal hyperexcitability following chronic ethanol abuse. The slight increase in *c-fos* expression observed in the hippocampus and cerebellum following acamprosate administration may reflect the increase in the NMDA component of excitatory transmission in these structures.

Rats from different strains (including various alcohol-preferring strains) were chronically treated with alcohol to study the EAA receptor subunit expression during various time intervals before and after withdrawal (Putzke et al. 1995). Our studies using in situ or dot blot hybridization in various brain structures illustrate that long-term ethanol consumption and ethanol withdrawal affects the expression of alternatively spliced messenger RNA encoding NMDARl receptor subunit variants. These experiments revealed marked differences in abundance and distribution of splice variant mRNA between ethanol-naive rats and animals which chronically ingest ethanol or undergo withdrawal. Following chronic ethanol consumption the levels of different

NMDARl splice variant mRNA decreased or remained unaltered in different brain structures. During ethanol withdrawal an elevation of several NMDARl splice variant mRNAs, for example, the NMDARl-4 variant (both deletions at the carboxy-terminal), were observed. The splice variants of the NMDAl receptor differ in their number of phosphorylation sites and ligand-binding properties. There is evidence that the degree of phosphorylation of NMDA receptor subunits alters the kinetics of the NMDA-activated channel (Westbrook 1994; Hollmann and Heinemann 1994).

Alterations of Behavior Induced by Acamprosate

Rats which were deprived of alcohol for 3 days after 8 months of continuous alcohol access increase their ethanol consumption after this deprivation phase. When acamprosate (50–200 mg/kg i.p.) was administered twice daily, alcohol-drinking following an alcohol-deprivation phase was decreased dose-dependently or even dropped below baseline drinking (Spanagel et al. 1996a). A radio telemetric system, which enabled us to monitor body temperature, locomotor activity, and food and water intake patterns constantly during alcohol withdrawal, was used for the quantification of alcohol withdrawal. Acamprosate given twice a day (200 mg/kg, i.p., 8 AM and 8 PM) reduced hyperlocomotion and food intake significantly in the alcohol withdrawal animals but did not change withdrawal-induced hyperthermia. When acamprosate was given to alcohol-naive animals, it transiently increased locomotor activity and body temperature, in particular during the rats' active night phase (Spanagel et al. 1996a). The results of generalization testing revealed that acamprosate failed to substitute for the ethanol cue whereas, in comparison, the non-competitive NMDA receptor antagonist dizocilpine (0.01 - 0.2 mg/kg i.p.) completely generalized for the ethanol cue (ED_{50} = 0.05 mg/kg). Acamprosate also had no effect when tested as an antagonist. Therefore neither the ethanol nor the saline discrimination was altered by acamprosate pretreatment. Furthermore, acamprosate had no effect on response latencies at any dose tested. These results suggest that this compound does not generalize for the ethanol cue and does not act as a substitution drug (Spanagel et al. 1996c).

Conclusion

Acamprosate probably interferes through various mechanisms with the altered excitability of central neurons resulting from chronic ethanol intake. Prominent sites of action of acamprosate are synaptic transmission which involves the activation of EAA receptors (Zeise et al. 1990, 1993; Zieglgänsberger and Zeise 1992; Berton et al. 1995; Madamba et al. 1995) and voltage-activated Ca^{2+} channels (Littleton et al. 1991). Through such actions acamprosate may counteract the long-lasting changes in neuronal excitability following chronic alcohol abuse which involve, for example, alterations in gene expression for EAA ion channel subunits, neuropeptides, intracellular regulators such as heat shock proteins, IEG-related transcription factors, and protein kinases or their ligands. Acamprosate, by preventing the expression of withdrawal in various neuronal systems, may interfere with synaptic plasticity related to the development and maintenance of addiction.

References

Berton F, Francesconi W, Madamba S, Zieglgänsberger W, Siggins GR (1995) The anti-craving agent acamprosate enhances NMDA-mediated EPSPs in rat nucleus accumbens in vitro. Soc Neurosci Abstr 21: 2101

Boismare F, Daoust M, Lhuintre JP, Ladure P, Rinjard P (1984) Are gamma aminobutyric acidergic receptors involved in the voluntary intake of ethanol by rats? J Pharmacol 15: 457–458

Boismare F, Daoust M, Moore N, Saligaut C, Lhuintre JP, Chretien P, Durlach J (1984b) A homotaurine derivate reduces the voluntary intake of ethanol by rats: are cerebral GABA receptors involved? Pharmacol Biochem Behav 21: 787–789

Boismare F, Daoust M, Lhuintre JP, Moore N, Saligaut C, Flipo JL (1986) Which GABA receptors are involved in the voluntary ethanol intake by rats? Alcohol Alcohol 21: A30 1986,

Daoust M, Legrand E, Gewiss M, Heidbreder C, DeWitte P, Tran G, Durbin P (1992) Acamprosate modulates synaptosomal GABA transmission in chronically alcoholised rats. Pharmacol Biochem Behav 41: 669–674

Gewiss M, Heidbreder C, Opsomer L, Durbin P, De Witte P (1991) Acamprosate and diazepam differentially modulate alcohol-induced behavioural and cortical alterations in rats following chronic inhalation of ethanol vapour. Alcohol Alcohol 26: 129–137

Guppy LJ, Littleton JM (1994) Binding characteristics of the calcium channel antagonist 3[H]-nitrendipine in tissue from ethanol-dependent rats. Alcohol Alcohol 29: 283–293

Hoffman PL, Tabakoff B (1994) The role of the NMDA receptor in ethanol withdrawal. In: Jansson B, Jörnvall H, Tydberg U, Terenius L, Vallee BL (eds) Toward a molecular basis of alcohol use and abuse. Birkhäuser, Basel, pp 61–70

Hollmann M, Heinemann S (1994) Cloned glutamate receptors. Annu Rev Neurosci 17: 31–108

Hunt SP, McNaughton LA, Jenkins R, Wisden W (1995) Immediate-early gene activation as a window on mechanism in the nervous system. In: Tölle TR, Schadrack J, Zieglgänsberger W (eds) Immediate-early genes in the central nervous system. Springer, Berlin Heidelberg New York pp 18–34

Kalant H (1993) Problems in the search for mechanisms of tolerance. Alcohol Alcohol [suppl] 2: 1–8

Ladewig D, Knecht T, Leher P, Fendl A (1993) Acamprosate – a stabilizing factor in long-term withdrawal of alcoholic patients. Ther Umschau 50: 182–188

Le Magnen J, Tran G, Durlach J (1987) Dose-dependent suppression of the high alcohol intake of chronically intoxicated rats by Ca-acetylhomotaurinate. Alcohol 4: 97–102

Lhuintre JP, Daoust M, Moore N, Chretien P, Saligaut C, Tran G, Boismare F, Jillemand B (1985) Ability of calcium bis acetyl homotaurine, a GABA agonist, to prevent relapse in weaned alcoholics. Lancet l: 1014–1016

Lhuintre JP, Moore N, Tran G, Steru L, Lancrenon S, Daoust M, Parot P, Ladure P, Zarnitsky C, Boismare F, Hillemand B (1990) Acamprosate appears to decrease alcohol intake in weaned alcoholics. Alcohol 25: 613–622

Littleton JM, Little H (1994) Current concepts of ethanol dependence. Addiction 89: 1397–1412

Littleton JM, Brennan C, Bouchenafa O (1991) The role of calcium flux in the central nervous system actions of ethanol. Ann NY Acad Sci 625: 388–394

Lovinger DM, White G, Weight FF (1989) Ethanol inhibits NMDA-activated ion currents in hippocampal neurons. Science 243: 1721–1724

Madamba SG, Schweitzer P, Zieglgänsberger W, Siggins GR (1995) Acamprosate (calcium acetylhomotaurinate) enhances the N-methyl-D-aspartate component of excitatory neurotransmission in rat hippocampal CA1 neurons in vitro. Alcohol Clin Exp Res (in press)

Nie Z, Yaun X, Madamba SG, Siggins GR (1993) Ethanol decreases glutamatergic synaptic transmission in rat nucleus accumbens in vitro: naloxone reversal. J Pharmacol Exp Ther 270: 1705–1712

Nie Z, Madamba SG, Siggins GR (1994) Ethanol inhibits glutamatergic neurotransmission in nucleus accumbens neurons by multople mechanisms. J Pharmacol Exp Ther 271: 1566–1573

Proctor WR, Dunwiddie TV (1991) Differential effects of ethanol on hippocampal cerebellar and cortical neurons from rat brain slices. Alcohol Clin Exp Res 15: 325
Proctor WR, Allan AM, Dunwiddie TV (1992) Brain region-dependent sensitivity of GABAa receptor-mediated responses to modulation by ethanol. Alcohol Clin Exp Res 16: 480–489
Putzke J, Spanagel R, Tölle TR, Zieglgänsberger W (1995) Differential expression of NMDARI splice variant mRNA in the brain of alcohol preferring rats with and without ethanol withdrawal. Pharmacopsychiatry 28: 205
Putzke J, Spanagel R, Tölle TR, Zieglgänsberger, W (1996) The anti-craving drug acamprosate reduces c-fos expression in rat undergoing ethanol withdrawal Eur J Pharmacol (in press)
Samson HH, Harris RA (1992) Neurobiology of alcohol abuse. Trends Neurosci 13: 206–211
Sanna E, Serra M, Cossu A, Colombo G, Follesa P, Cuccheddu T, Concas A, Biggio G (1993) Chronic ethanol intoxication induces differential effects on $GABA_A$ and NMDA receptor function in the rat brain. Alcohol Clin Exp Res 17: 115–123
Siggins GR, Pittman Q, French E (1987) Effects of ethanol on CA1 and CA3 pyramidal cells in the hippocampal slice preparation: an intracellular study. Brain Res 414: 22–34
Soldo BL, Proctor WR, Dunwiddie TV (1994) Ethanol differentially modulates GABAA receptor-mediated chloride currents in hippocampal, cortical, and septal neurons in rat brain slices. Synapse 18: 94–103
Spanagel R, Hölter SM, Allingham K, Landgraf R, Zieglgänsberger W (1996a) Acamprosate and alcohol. I. Effects on reinstatement behaviour in the alcohol-dependent rat. Eur J Pharmacol (in press)
Spanagel R, Putzke J, Stefferl A, Schöbitz B, Zieglgänsberger W (1996b) Acamprosate and alcohol. II. Effects on alcohol withdrawal. Eur J Pharmacol (in press)
Spanagel R, Zieglgänsberger W, Hundt W (1996c) Acamprosate and alcohol. III. Effects on alcohol discrimination. Eur J Pharmacol (in press)
Westbrook GL Glutamate receptor update. Curr Opin Neurobiol 4: 1994, 337-346
Wisden W, Seeburg PH Mammalian ionotropic glutamate receptors. Curr Opin Neurobiol: 291–298
Zeise ML, Kasparow S, Capogna M, Zieglgänsberger W (1990) Calciumdiacetyl-homotaurinate (Ca-AOTA) decreases the action of excitatory amino acids in the rat neocortex in vitro. Prog Clin Biol Res 351: 237–242
Zeise ML, Kasparow S, Capogna M, Zieglgänsberger W (1993) Calcium diacetyl-homotaurinate (Ca-AOTA) decreases the action of excitatory amino acids in the rat neocortex in vitro, Eur J Pharmacol 231: 47–52
Zieglgänsberger W, Zeise ML (1992) Calcium-diacetyl-homotaurinate which prevents relapse in weaned alcoholics decreases the action of excitatory amino acids in neocortical neurons of the rat in vitro. In: Naranjo CS, Sellers EM (eds) Novel pharmacological interventions for alcoholism. Springer, Berlin Heidelberg New York, pp 337–341
Zieglgänsberger W, Hauser C, Putzke J, Spanagel R, Wetzel C (1995) The enhanced excitability of central neurons following chronic alcohol intake is reduced by Acamprosate. Alcohol Alcohol 30: 552

Acamprosate Decreases Alcohol Behavioral Dependence and Hypermotility After Alcohol Withdrawal But Increases Inhibitory Amino-Acids in Alcohol-Attracted Inbred Rats Using Microdialysis of the Nucleus Accumbens

P. De Witte[1], A. Dahchour[1], E. Quertemont [1], P. Durbin[2], and S. Chabac[2]

Introduction

Evidence from neurochemical, behavioral, and binding studies increasingly points to neuroexcitatory and neuroinhibitory amino-acids as being of fundamental importance in mediating the effects of ethanol drinking behavior. We therefore investigated the respective effects of increasing doses of acamprosate, an acetylated form of homotaurine salified by Ca^{2+}, on blood alcohol level, on the alcohol-induced hypermotility of the animals during the withdrawal syndrome, and on dependence towards alcohol. We also examined the effects of acamprosate on the extracellular concentration of excitatory and inhibitory amino acids in the nucleus accumbens in vivo. The nucleus accumbens appears to be essential in the regulation of motivated behaviors, particularly in the rewarding properties of a variety of abused substances, including ethanol.

Materials and Methods

Subjects

Two hundred adult male rats of the Wistar strain were housed individually in plexiglass breeding cages throughout the experiment. Food and water were available ad libitum. At the time of the experiments body weights ranged from 300 to 350 g. Animals were anesthetized with chloral hydrate (400 mg/kg, IP) and received maintenance doses each hour to maintain a constant level of anesthesia throughout the experiment. Each rat was mounted in a stereotaxic

[1]Laboratory Psychobiology, University of Louvain, 1 Place Croix-du-Sud, 1348 Louvain-la-Neuve, Belgium
[2]Groupe LIPHA, Campral International Product Management, 34, rue St. Romain, 69379 Lyon Cedex 8, France

frame with the upper incisor bar set 3.5 mm below the interaural line. The skull was exposed, and a hole was drilled for unilateral placement of the dialysis probe, which was implanted into the nucleus accumbens according to the following coordinates: A-P 1.2 mm; L 1.2 mm; V 6.7 mm.

Selection of Alcohol-Attracted and Alcohol-NonAttracted Inbred Rats

Each Wistar inbred rat was offered two bottles, one containing top water and the other 10% (v/v) ethanol for 1 week. Ethanol alcohol-attracted (AA) rats consumed at least 20% of the offered 10% ethanol drinking bottle in a free-choice situation while alcohol-nonattracted (ANA) rats took more than 90% of the fluid intake at the water drinking bottle. We started this selection with 200 rats and obtained finally 10 AA rats (5%) and 12 ANA rats (6%). AA and ANA rats were than divided into two groups each. The control group (6ANA, 5A) received one bottle containing tap water and were housed individually for 4 weeks before receiving an IP injection of 15% ethanol (2 g/kg) before microdialysis began. The treated group (6ANA, 5A) received one bottle containing water to which was added acamprosate (400 mg/kg per day) and were housed individually for 4 weeks before receiving an IP injection of 15% ethanol (2 g/kg) before microdialysis began.

Brain Microdialysis Procedure

The dialysis probes were constructed as described by Robinson and Whishaw (1988). Dialysis tubing extended 3 mm beyond the tip of the probe. The probe was connected to a microinfusion pump, continuously perfused at 1 μl/min with Ringer's solution. Perfusates were collected every 20 min in microcentrifuges tubes connected to the outlet cannula. Each tube contained 10 μl 0.1 m*M* EDTA to prevent air oxidation and 10 μl 5 μ*M* N^{G}-nitro-L-arginine as internal standard. Once amino acid levels in the perfusates had stabilized (80–100 mm), six consecutive samples were collected every 20 min for the determination of basal levels. Rats were then injected IP with an equal volume of either saline or 15% (v/v) ethanol (1, 2, or 3 g/kg body weight) in 0.9% saline and 20-min dialysis samples were collected for another 120 min. A sample of 20 rats received an IP injection of 1 g/kg acamprosate before microdialysis of the nucleus accumbens to estimate the effect of acamprosate on the accumbal amino-acids. Another sample of 20 rats received 400 mg/kg acamprosate per os daily for 30 days in their drinking bottles before an IP injection of 2 g/kg ethanol; the nucleus accumbens was then dialysated for quantification of the amino-acids.

For chronic treatment naive rats were divided into groups receiving daily two IP injections of 15% ethanol (v/v) or saline 0.9%: 1 g/kg ethanol for 1 week followed by 2 g/kg the 2 week before microdialysis. The same procedure used as for acute injection was then followed, i.e., IP injection of an equal volume of saline or 15% (v/v) ethanol followed by 20-min dialysis samples collected for another 120 min.

Simultaneous Determination of Excitatory and Inhibitory Amino Acids

The concentration of amino acids was determined using HPLC-EC following precolumn *O*-phtaldialdehyde (OPA) derivatization. After 27 mg OPA was disolved in 1 ml methanol HPLC-grade with 10 $\mu l/\beta$-mercaptoethanol (BME), this solution was diluted with 9 ml 0.1 *M* sodium tetraborate buffer, pH 9.3, and stored at 4° C. The working solution was prepared each day, 24 h before use, by diluting 1 ml of the above solution in 3 ml 0.1 *M* sodium tetraborate. The derivatization procedure entailed mixing the dialysate and the internal standard with 10 µl OPA/BME for 2 min in complete darkness before injection into the HPLC system. This system consisted of a ConstaMetric pump delivering 1 ml/min of the mobile phase at a pressure of 5300 psi. Separation of amino-acids was achieved with reversed-phase column (100 × 3.2 Biophase-II, ODS 3 µm) and detected coulometrically using three electrodes: a guard (0.4 V), preoxidation (-0.4 V), and working (+0.6 V) electrode (Donzanti and Yamamoto 1988). The mobile phase used (0.1 *M* Na_2HPO_4, × 13.4 m*M* EDTA, × 32% methanol HPLC grade, 68% Milliq H_2O, pH 6.4) was filtered through 0.2-µm cellulose nitrate filter and degassed under vacuum before use in the HPLC system. The position and height of peaks of the endogenous components were compared with a standard solution prepared from a 10^{-3} *M* concentration of aspartate, glutamate, taurine, and GABA in a solution of Milliq water and HPLC-grade methanol. The working solution was prepared each day by diluting 10^{-3}–10^{-6} *M* in Ringer's solution, and 20-µl samples of this solution were injected and quantified by PC integration pack.

Chronic Alcohol Intoxication

The animals, individually housed, were maintained for 30 days in an isolated plastic chamber (160 × 60 × 60 cm) in an alcohol-containing atmosphere. A mixture of alcohol and air was pulsed into the chamber via a mixing system allowing the quantity of alcohol to be increased every 2 days during the entire experimental procedure. The animals were kept for 30 days in the alcoholization chamber. One hundred adult rats were randomly divided into five experimental groups of 20 rats each: the first group had free access to water (control group) while the other four groups received acamprosate in their drinking bottle 50, 100, 200, on 400 mg/kg/per day) during the entire alcoholization procedure (30 days). The control group was used to determine the level of behavioral dependence without acamprosate treatment. In the treated groups no further acamprosate was diluted in the drinking bottles once the pulmonary alcoholization ended.

Blood Alcohol Level

The blood alcohol level was determined regularly in each of the five groups throughout the period of alcoholization exposure (30 days) in 0.1-ml samples obtained from the caudal portion of the tail according to an alcohol dehydrogenase method (Boehringer-Mannheim kit).

Motility Recording

To study hypermotility during the withdrawal syndrome after the 4-week alcoholization period ten rats treated with acamprosate (50 mg/kg per day) and ten untreated animals were placed for 18 h in an apparatus designed to detect motility operating on to the principle of inertia. Movements of animals were transmitted to a plate supported by steel balls with minimal resistance.

Free-Choice Paradigm

At the end of the 4-week-alcoholization period control and treated rats were submitted to three successive steps: (a) full beverage deprivation (the last 18 h of the alcohol intoxication period and the first 6 h of the withdrawal period), (b) presentation of a 10% (v/v) ethanol solution as the sole drinking fluid during the following 18 h and (c) a free-choice beverage situation [water vs a 10% (v/v) ethanol solution] for a period of 30 days. During the free choice period fluid consumption was recorded daily.

Data Analyses

Neurochemical dose-response data were transformed into data points representing the average of the last three 20 microdialysis samples for each dose and then analyzed by a two-way analysis of variance (treatment group × time) with repeated measures on one factor, followed by the least significant difference test of multiple comparison (Fisher's test) to determine statistical significance between treatment and control values. Data from motility recording were analyzed using analyses of variance for repeated measures (general linear models procedure).

Results

Microdialysis

Acute Effects of Ethanol

Figure 1 shows the effects of acute ethanol and saline IP injections on the extracellular concentrations of glutamate, taurine, and GABA. Acute ethanol induced a rapid and significant increase only in taurine concentration, ethanol failed to modify the extracellular glutamate and GABA concentrations in the microdialysate from the nucleus accumbens.

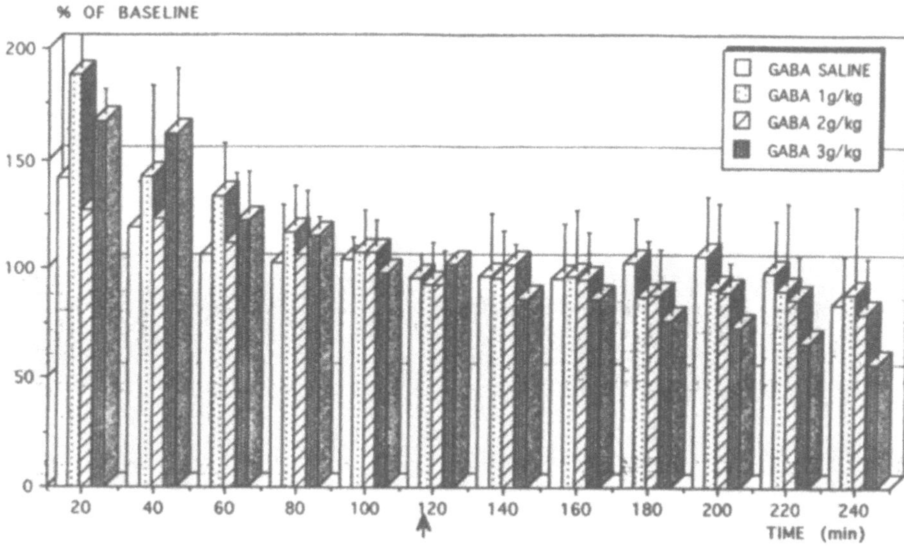

a

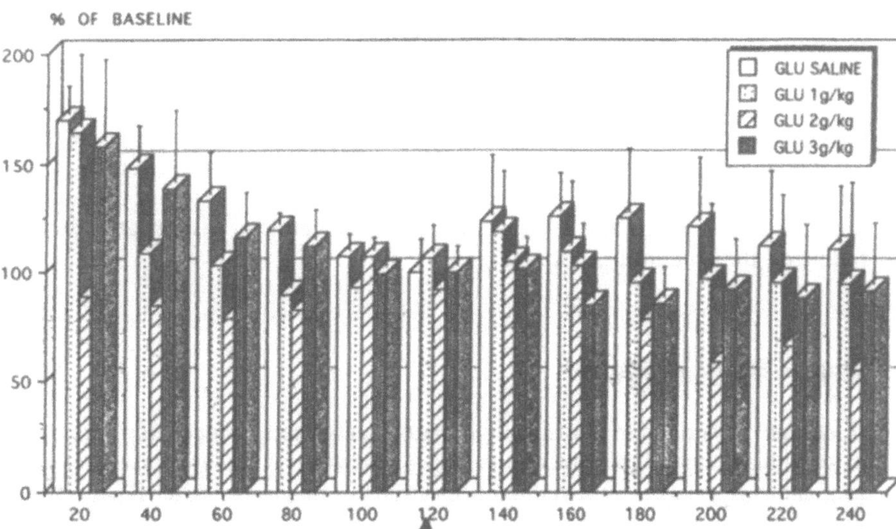

b

Fig. 1a-c. Effects of acute IP injection of ethanol (1,2,3 g/kg body weight) on extracellular GABA, glutamate (*GLU*), and taurine (*TAU*) content of the microdialysate from the nucleus accumbens. $^*p < 0.05$ vs. baseline.

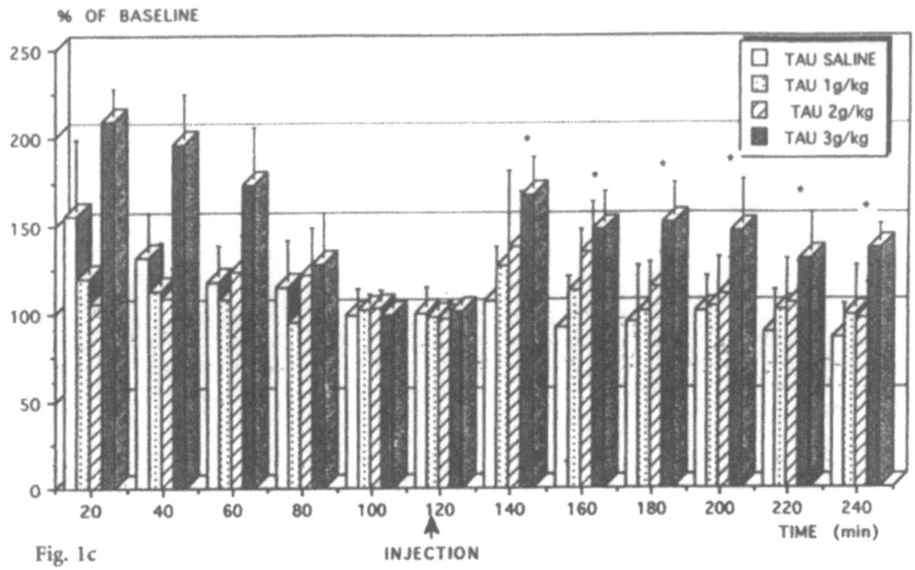

Fig. 1c

Acamprosate IP Injections and Pretreatment

The IP injection of acamprosate induced modifications in the extracellular concentration only in taurine; the significant increase of taurine lasted at least 3 h following the injection (Fig. 2). Pretreatment with acamprosate orally for 30 days in the drinking bottle at 400 mg/kg induced a potentiation of the taurine increase produced by the IP injection of 3 g/kg ethanol lasting at least 3 h following the ethanol injection (Fig. 3).

Chronic Effects of Ethanol

IP ethanol injections in chronically ethanol treated rats induced an increase in extracellular taurine concentrations (Fig. 4). However, these increases were not as great as those after acute ethanol injections in naive rats. After IP injections of 1 g/kg ethanol there was a slight but nonsignificant increase in the taurine concentration. Again, none of the tested doses of ethanol modified the extracellular glutamate and GABA concentrations (Fig. 4).

Effect of Acute Ethanol in AA Rats and ANA Rats

After a single IP dose of ethanol (2 g/kg) to AA and ANA rats there was a significant change in extracellular taurine content only in the ANA rats. No changes occurred in the AA rats in any of the amino-acids tested (Fig. 5).

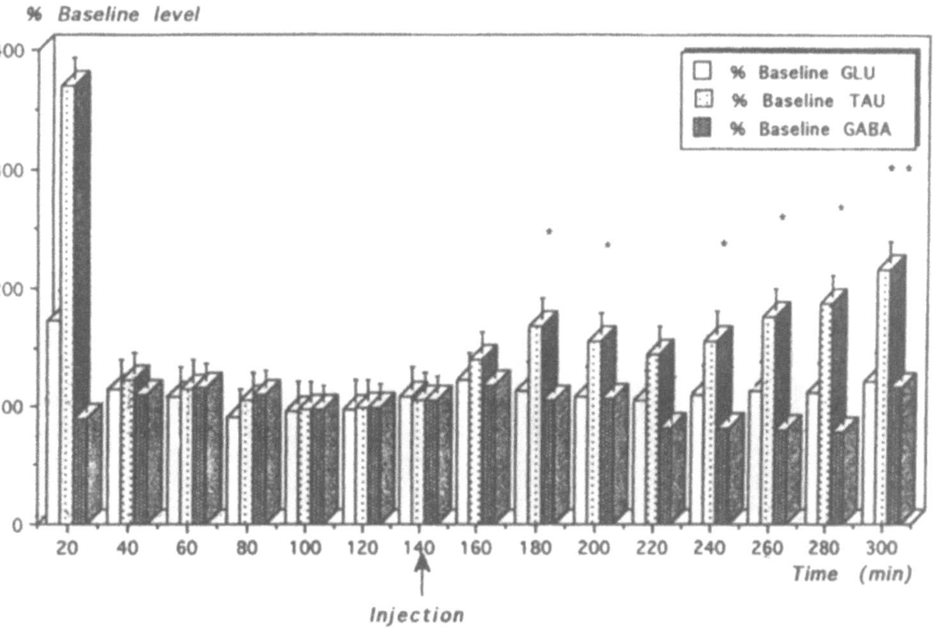

Fig. 2. Increase in taurine (*TAU*) but not glutamate (*GLU*) nor GABA after an IP injection of acamprosate (1 g/kg). * $p < 0.05$; ** $p < 0.01$ vs. baseline

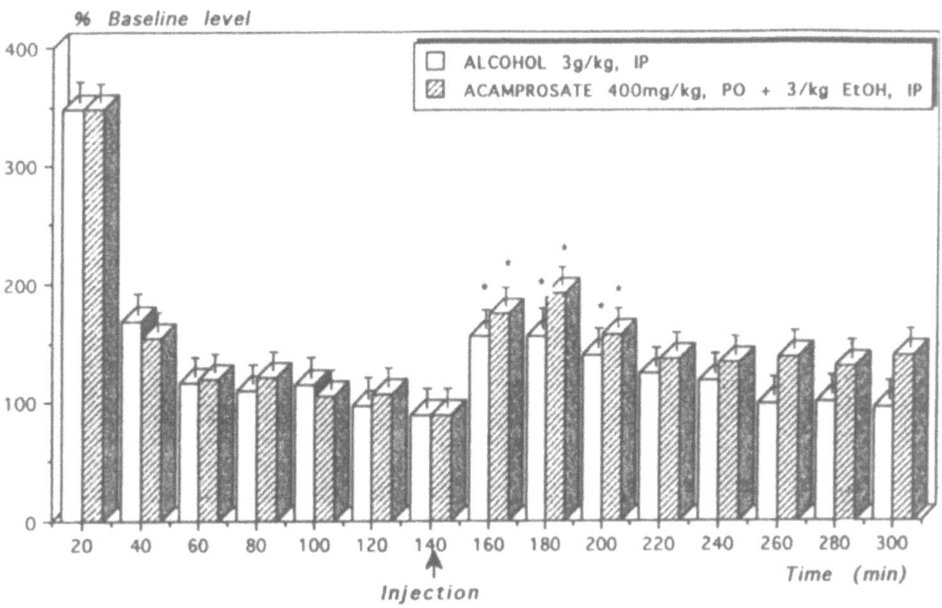

Fig. 3. Potentiation of the extracellular accumbal taurine by pretreatment with acamprosate (400 mg/kg PO) followed by an acute injection of alcohol (3 kg/kg IP). * $p < 0.05$ vs. baseline

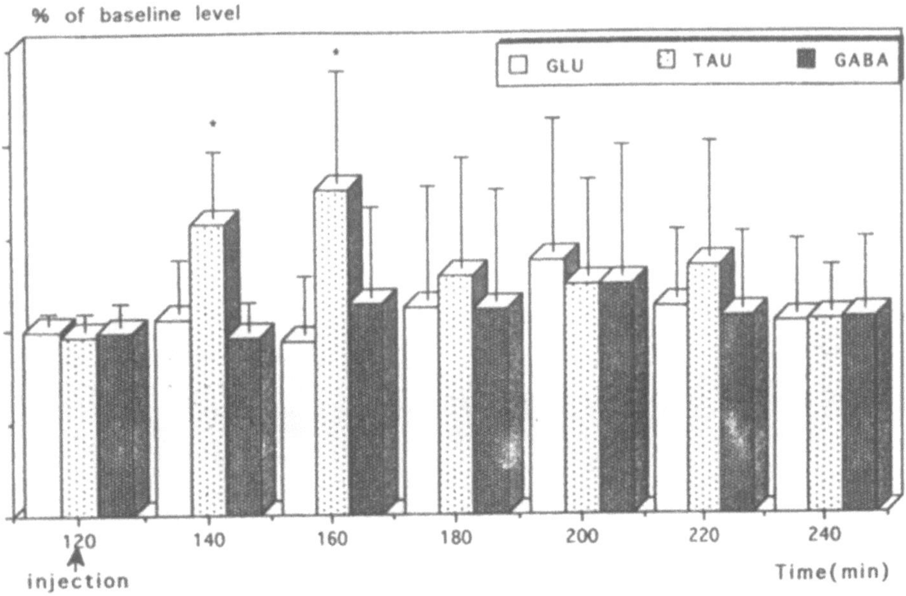

Fig. 4. Effects of an acute injection of 2 g/kg ethanol on the extracellular glutamate (*GLU*), taurine (*TAU*) and GABA in the accumbens of chronically ethanol-treated rats.* $p < 0.05$ vs. baseline

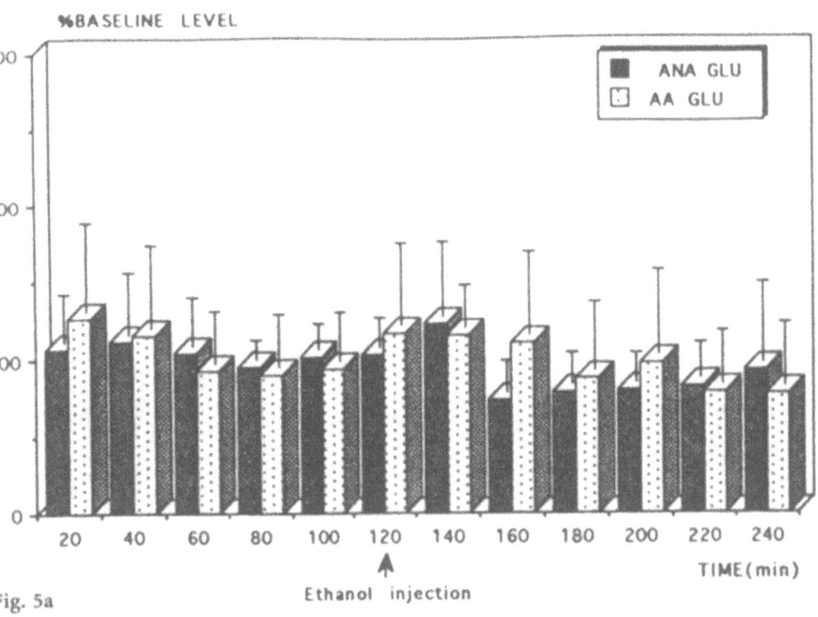

Fig. 5a

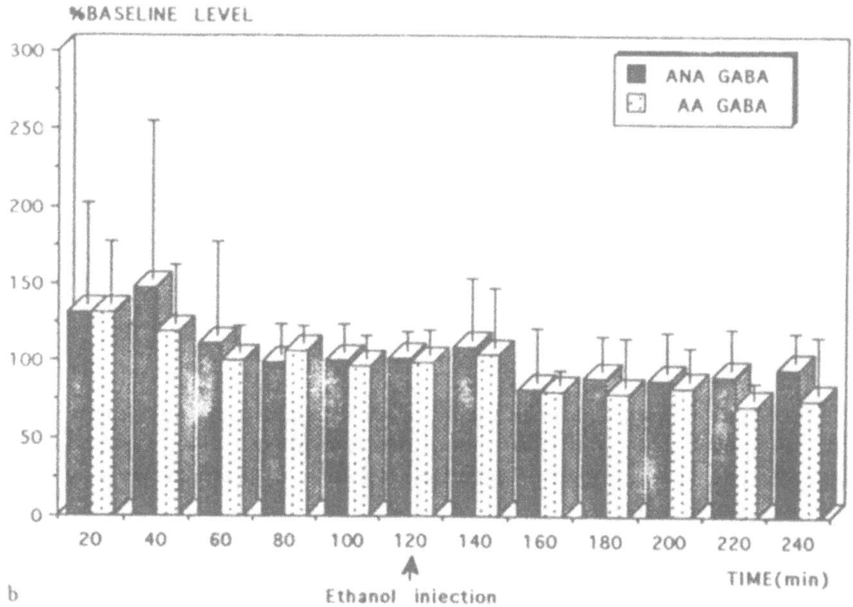

b

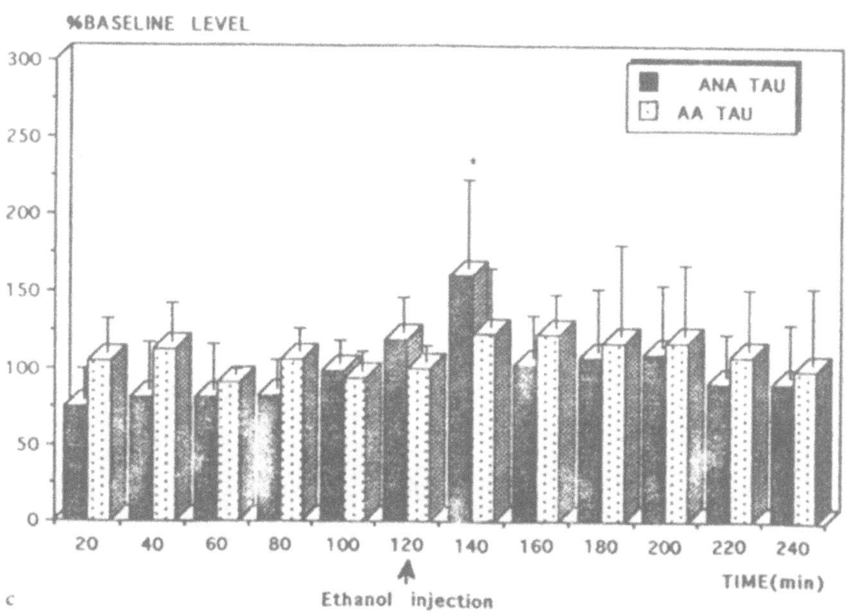

c

Fig. 5a-c. Effects of an acute injection of 2 g/kg ethanol on extracellular glutamate, GABA and taurine (*TAU*) in AA and ANA rats. Only taurine was increased in the ANA rats. * $p < 0.05$ vs. baseline

Effect of Acute Ethanol in AA Rats and ANA Rats Pretreated with Acamprosate

After a single IP dose of ethanol (2 g/kg) the taurine content of the microdialysate from both AA and ANA increased and was similar after acamprosate administration (Fig. 6a). Glutamate increased in the AA group after 100 min (Fig. 6b) while Gaba decreased after 20 min for a duration of a least 120 min postinjection (Fig. 6c) No changes, other than taurine, occurred in the ANA group following a pretreatment of acamprosate.

Blood Alcohol Level

The spectrophotometric assay of the blood alcohol level and a linear regression analysis showed that the alcoholemia of rats treated with acamprosate did not significantly differ from that of untreated rats for any treatment considered in these experiments (Fig. 7).

Motility Recording

As shown in Fig. 8, hypermotility was observed in alcoholized untreated rats for approximately 10 h following the 4-week alcoholization period. Acamprosate (50 mg/kg) immediately reduced this hyperactivity.

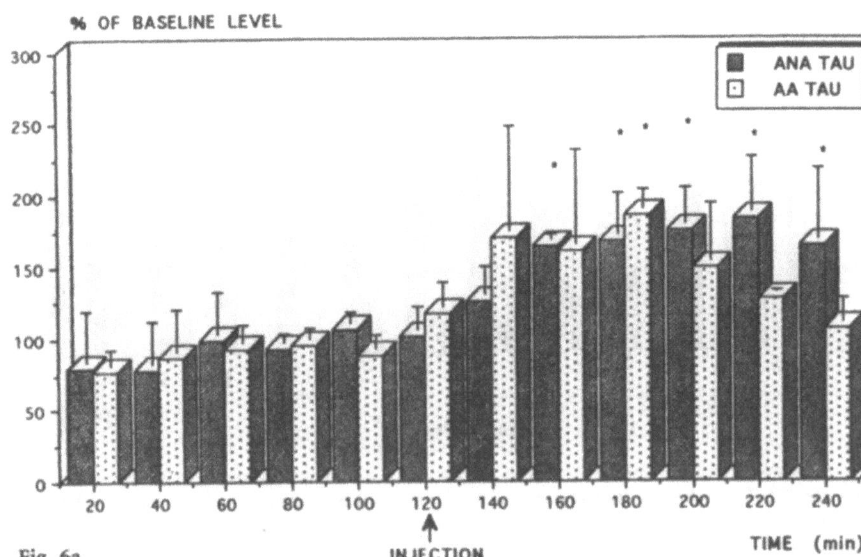

Fig. 6a

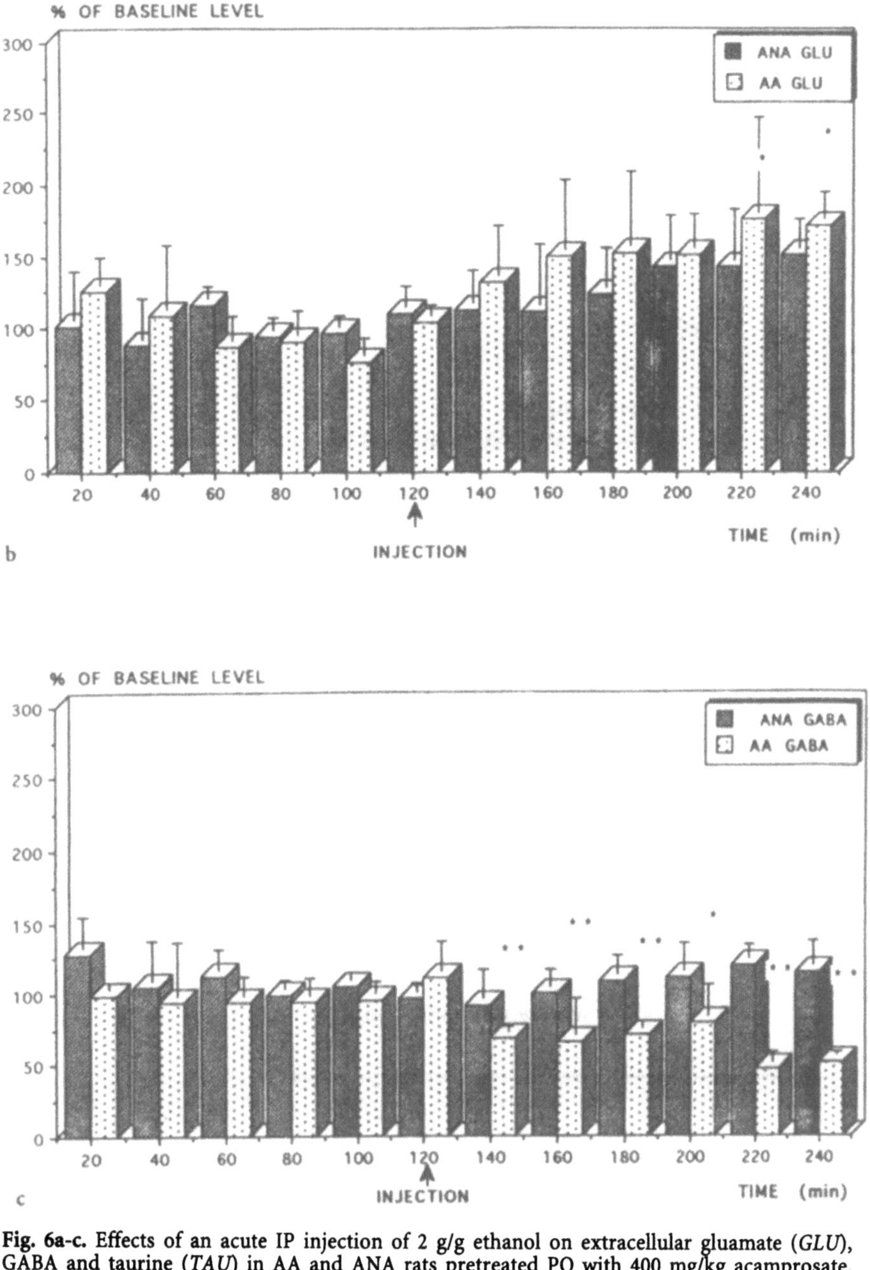

Fig. 6a-c. Effects of an acute IP injection of 2 g/g ethanol on extracellular gluamate (*GLU*), GABA and taurine (*TAU*) in AA and ANA rats pretreated PO with 400 mg/kg acamprosate. Taurine increased in both AA and ANA rats while glutamate increased late only in the AA rats, together with a decrease in GABA in the same AA rats. * $p < 0.05$; ** $p < 0.01$ vs. baseline

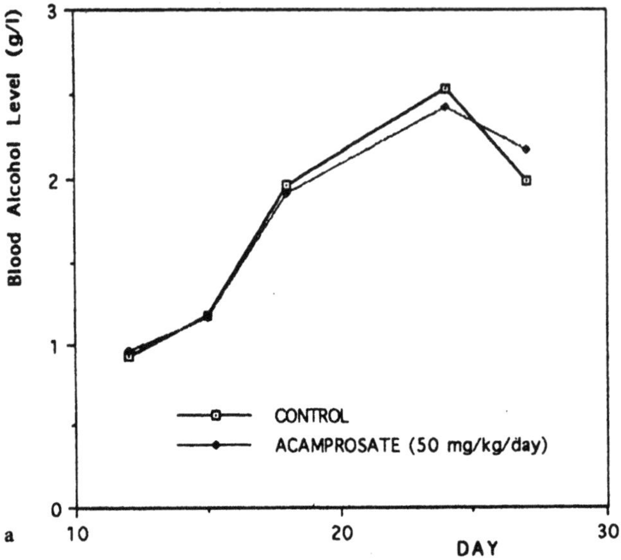

a

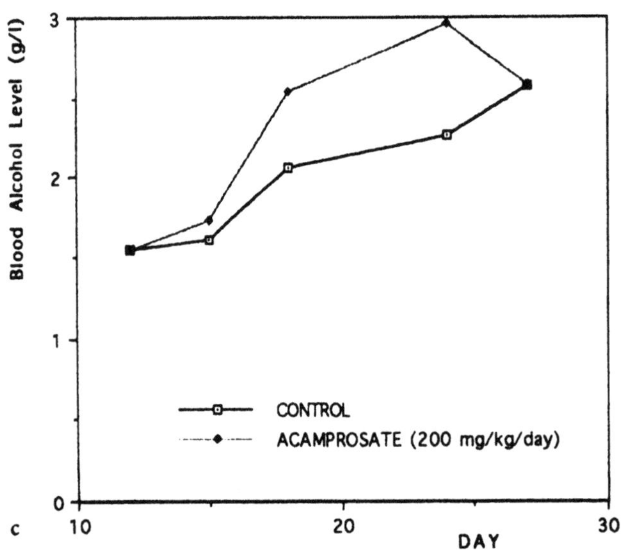

c

Fig. 7a-d. Blood alcohol level of control and acamprosate - treated rats during pulmonary alcoholization. Blood samples were analyzed from day 12th after the onset of chronic alcohol intoxication

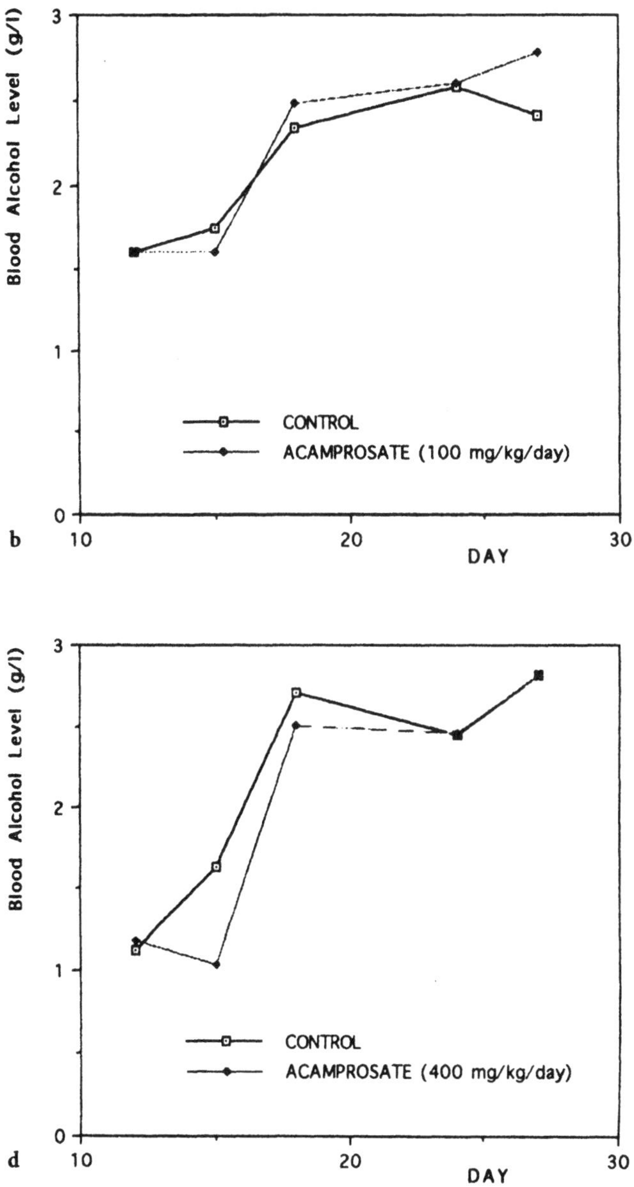
Blood Alcohol Level (g/l)
3
2
1
0
CONTROL
ACAMPROSATE (100 mg/kg/day)
b
10
20
30
DAY
Blood Alcohol Level (g/l)
3
2
1
0
CONTROL
ACAMPROSATE (400 mg/kg/day)
d
10
20
30
DAY

Fig. 7b,d

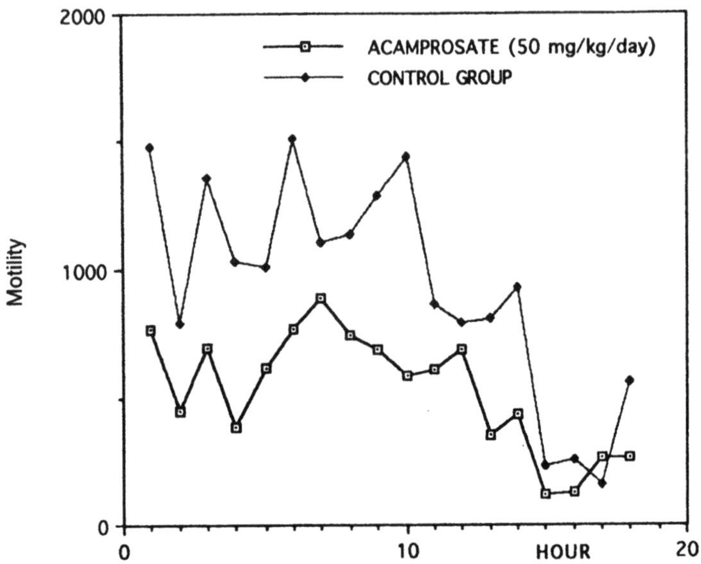

Fig. 8. Spontaneous motor activity. Recording of the hypermotility observed during the withdrawal syndrome in control and acamprosate pulmonary alcoholized rats. *Abscissa*, time sequence after a 4-week alcoholization period

Free-Choice Paradigm

In free-choice paradigm experiment performed at the end of the chronic alcoholization study, untreated rats displayed preference to alcohol, as expressed by a greater alcohol consumption than water intake during the first 23 days (Fig. 9a). Interestingly, increasing doses of acamprosate (50, 100, 200 mg/kg) progressively reduced this preference for alcohol (Fig. 9b-d). While acamprosate (50 mg/kg) did not reduce alcohol overconsumption during the first 23 days (no difference to untreated rats), the difference between the two curves remained significant for 13 days after acamprosate at 100 mg/kg (Fig. 9c) and for 11 days after acamprosate at 200 mg/kg (Fig. 9d). Finally, acamprosate at 400 mg/kg immediately abolished the preference for alcohol (Fig. 9e, 10).

Discussion

The nucleus accumbens is one of the most important structures that contributes to limbic-motor integration, thus playing a key role in translating the motivational determinants of behavior into actions. The nucleus accumbens has been shown to play an important role in mediating the reinforcing effects of a number of drugs including alcohol (Koob 1992). Amino-acids neurotransmitters could participate in the reinforcing properties of ethanol, probably through the potentiation of $GABA_A$ (Korpi 1994; Kuriyama and Ueha 1992) and $GABA_B$ (Mehta and Ticku 1990) receptors. The effects of GABAergic agents on

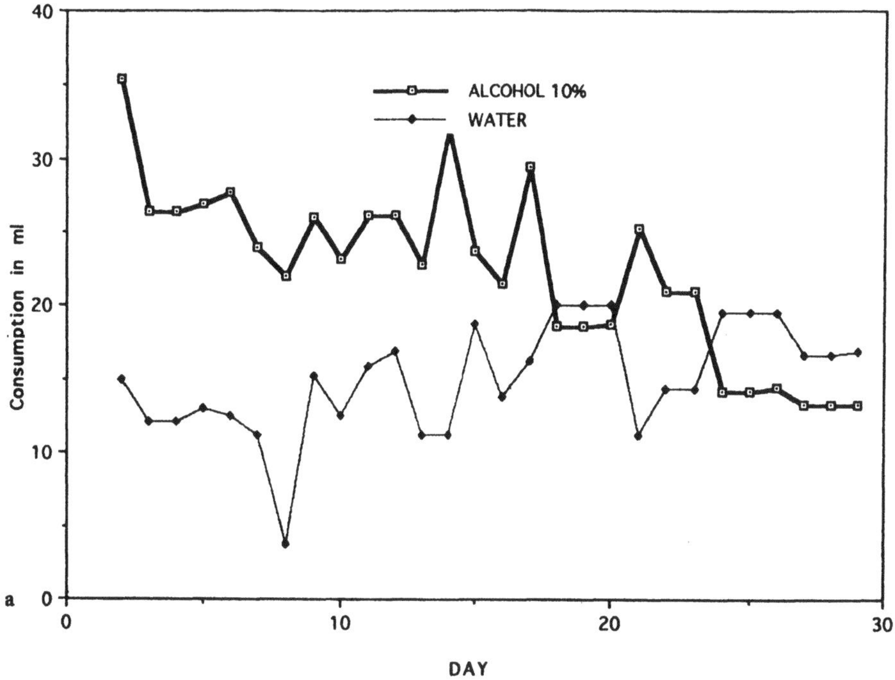

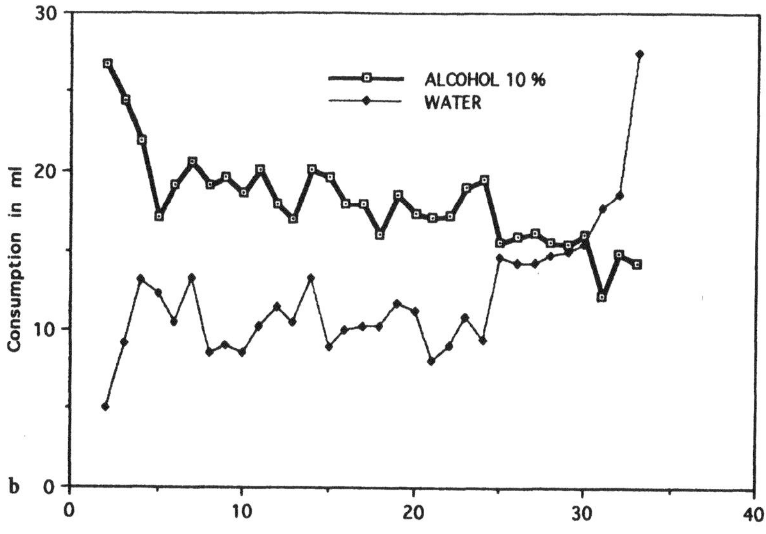

Fig. 9a-e. Alcohol and water consumption in pulmonary alcoholized untreated and acamprosate-treated rats as expressed in a free-choice beverage procedure. **a** control group. Acamprosate: **b** 50 mg/kg/day; **c** 100 mg/kg/day; **s** 200 mg/kg /day; **e** 400 mg/kg/day

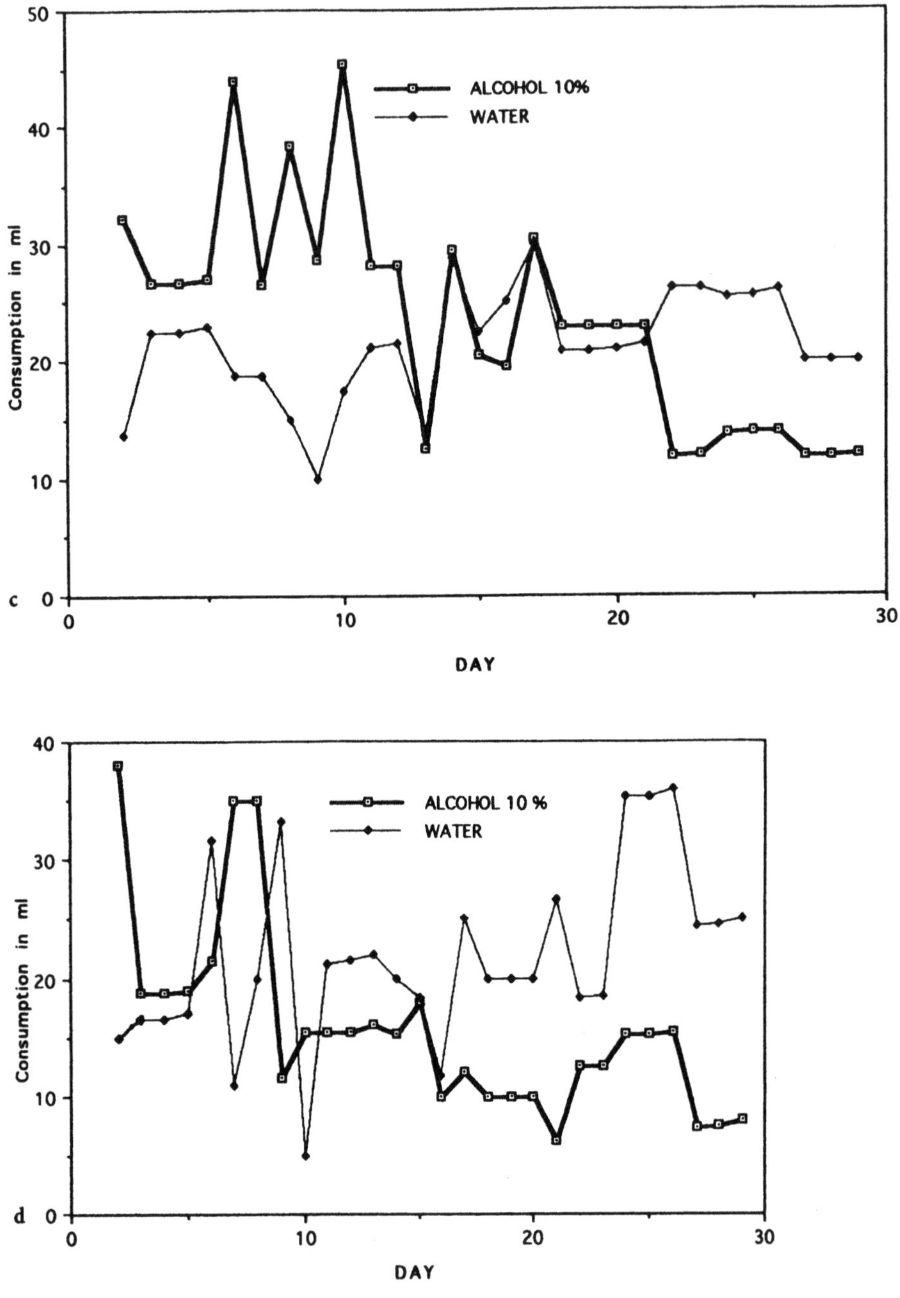

50
40
30
20
10
0
c
ALCOHOL 10%
WATER
Consumption in ml
0
10
20
30
DAY
40
30
20
10
0
d
ALCOHOL 10 %
WATER
Consumption in ml
0
10
20
30
DAY

Fig. 9c,d

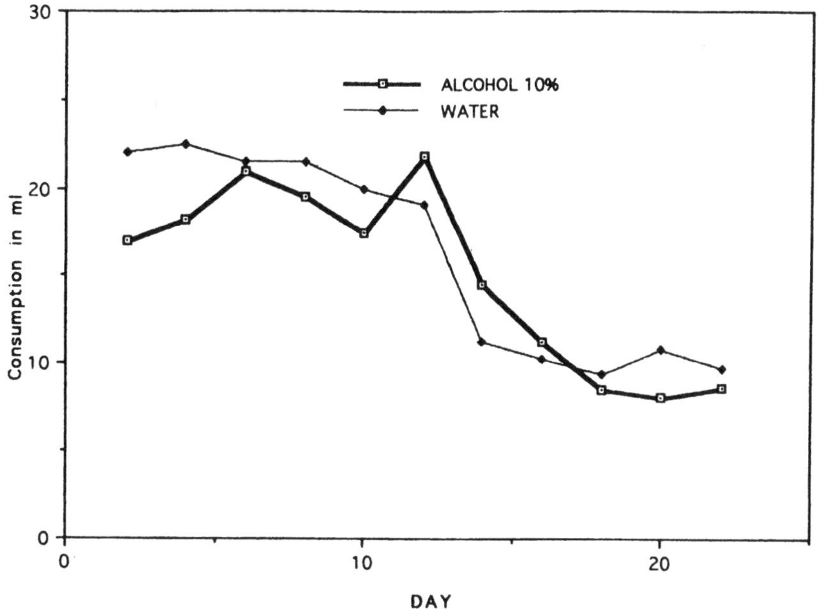

Fig. 9e

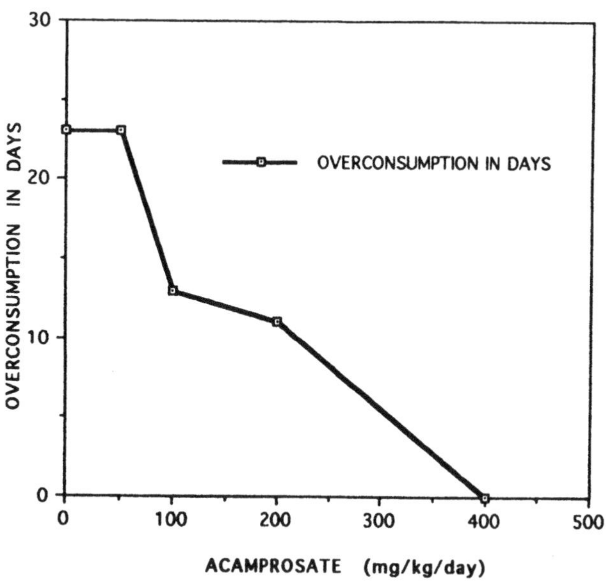

Fig. 10. Dependence towards alcohol: time of overconsumption

ethanol reinforcement have been studied extensively in several experiments, but the results have proven contradictory (Boyle et al. 1992; Rassnick et al. 1993; Smith et al. 1992). Excitatory amino-acids have also been implicated in the action of ethanol, particularly the *N*-Methyl-D-aspartate receptors (Deitrich et al. 1989; Weight et al. 1991; Lovinger et al. 1989).

The present study shows that acute and chronic ethanol produces a significant increase in the microdialysate extracellular taurine concentration without affecting the other amino acids. Although the microdialysis technique does not resolve the issue of the source of extracellular taurine increase, we can formulate several hypothesis:

1.Taurine could participate in the volume regulation of the brain nervous tissue disturbed by ethanol. Kimelberg et al. (1993) showed that incubation of primary astrocytes cultures with isosmotic ethanol causes cell swelling, leading to the release of taurine.

2.Taurine has also been shown to protect against oxidant-induced lung damage, possibly by reacting with hypochlorous acid to form *N*-chlorotaurine at the site of inflammation (Schuller-Levis et al. 1994). Nevertheless, no studies on the effect of taurine supplementation on alcohol-induced damage have been reported.

3.Taurine has also been suggested to increase the metabolic rate of ethanol (Iida and Hikichi 1976). However, no differences in blood ethanol were observed after taurine administration (Aragon et al. 1992).

4.Furthermore, taurine has been proposed to be an activator of the enzyme aldehyde dehydrogenase (Watanabe et al. 1985). Therefore taurine could reduce levels of the major metabolite of ethanol, acetaldehyde, which has been implicated in the development of both alcohol dependency (Von Wartburg and Bühler 1984) and tissue damage (Peters and Ward 1988).

5.Finally, it can be suggested that ethanol disturbs the assumed neurotransmitter or neuromodulatory function of taurine. Taurine may be implicated in some of the behavioral effects of ethanol. Several studies have reported that taurine exerts a significant effect on some ethanol-induced behaviors such as narcosis (Boggan et al. 1978), locomotor activity (Aragon et al. 1992), and conditioned taste aversion (Aragon and Amit 1993).

One of the ultimate aims of the present study was to identify the neurochemical basis for preferential alcohol intake in AA rats which could identify factors involved in the development of dependence and may eventually form the basis of treatment. A heterogeneous group of inbred rats was divided according to their attraction or nonattraction for alcohol. AA rats drank at least 20% of the ethanol solution offered in a free-choice situation with food and water available while ANA rats took more than 90% of water. This has been shown not to be a simple matter of taste preference as rats self-administered ethanol intragastrically (Waller et al. 1984). Moreover, AA rats increased their palatability after having access to alcohol since they associated the taste of alcohol with its positively reinforcing effects during free-access periods (Beeker et al. 1990). Reduced levels of dopamine have been observed in the nucleus accumbens of genetically bred alcohol-preferring rats (McBride et al. 1993) suggesting a deficit in the mesolimbic dopamine pathway projecting from the ventral tegmental area (VTA) which might be responsible for the higher consumption of alcohol. In addition, low serotonin levels in alcohol-preferring rats (Murphy 1987–1988) and high alcohol drinking rats (Cloninger 1987) may also promote alcohol intake. Indeed, administration of either a serotonin agonist or increasing the extracellular pool of serotonin or dopamine attenuates alcohol intake by alcohol-preferring rats.

In the nucleus accumbens the basal microdialysate content of the excitatory and inhibitory amino-acids was essentially similar in these two groups. After a single IP dose of ethanol (2 g/kg) to AA and ANA rats there was a significant change in the taurine content of the microdialysate only in the ANA, which showed the increase in taurine. In naive rats this increase in extracellular taurine concentration in the ANA group may exert some neuroprotective effect against alcohol toxicity. For example, it has been shown that preatreatment of rats with taurine prior to ethanol administration significantly reduces blood and liver acetaldehyde concentrations (Watanabe et al. 1985). ANA rats seem more sensitive to ethanol than AA rats as they present a higher enhancement in release of taurine after acute ethanol administration.

Effect of Ethanol in AA and ANA Rats Pretreated with Acamprosate

The taurine content of the microdialysate from the AA and ANA rats was similar after acamprosate but was significantly higher in the ANA. Since acamprosate is slowly degraded in vivo, it is unlikely that the increase in taurine comes from metabolism of the drug. Such changes in the taurine content could be related to increased neurosensitization to alcohol or to a consequence of its pharmacological actions, such that the more potent taurine-releasing effects in ANA than in AA rats may be one of the neurochemical basis of alcohol avoidance of the ANA group.

When the AA were challenged with an IP injection of ethanol (2 g/kg), there was a dramatic and immediate increase in the taurine level, which was sustained for a further 60 min, suggesting that acamprosate in some undefined way increases the neurosensitization to alcohol in the AA group. Furthermore, the extracellular concentration of GABA decreased after ethanol injection but only in the AA animals pretreated with acamprosate. It has been previously postulated that one of the mechanisms of action of acamprosate is related to $GABA_B$ receptors (Gewiss et al. 1991). Since there is strong evidence that the activation of $GABA_B$ autoreceptors depresses the release of GABA (Daoust et al. 1987; Bowery 1989), the increase in GABA in the microdialysate could represent an indirect effect induced by the late increase of glutamate after the ethanol injection observed in the AA group only.

Comparing the results in AA and ANA rats, both treated with acamprosate, we suggest that the release of taurine after acute administration of ethanol in the ANA group plays a major role in their avoidance of alcohol intake, supported by the fact that a greater increase in taurine was observed in rats pretreated with acamprosate. However, it is still unclear how and where taurine acts, as is the relationship between taurine and GABA and glutamate.

Concerning alcohol withdrawal and alcohol consumption, evidence suggests that the mechanisms of action of acamprosate are related more to GABAB receptors since these receptors are coupled to inhibition of Ca^{2+} channels in central neurons (Bowery 1989) and are stimulated by the GABAB receptor agonist baclofen, whose binding is modulated by divalent cations such as Ca^{2+} (Kato et al. 1982; Nanima et al. 1982).

Our results thus suggest that the acamprosate-induced suppression of the hypermotility produced by chronic alcoholization may be GABAB-dependent treatment. Interestingly, increasing dosages of acamprosate progressively reduced preference for alcohol whereas 400 mg/kg acamprosate per day completely prevented this behavior by balancing water and alcohol consumption. In the same way acamprosate administered orally to ethanol-naive rate over a 48-h period, has been show to enhance their spontaneous aversion to ethanol (Lhuintre et al. 1985).

The profiles described above on their own thus provide evidence that ethanol intake and alcohol withdrawal induce signs most probably related to distinct mechanisms which require specific treatments. Further steps must be taken to confirm or clarify the interaction between alcohol dependence, alcohol withdrawal, and amino-acids (neuroexcitatory and neuroinhibitory). Our data strongly suggest that acamprosate does not interfere with alcohol metabolism, but in a dose-related manner restricts the preference for alcohol in dependent animals and strongly erases the hyperactivation induced by the withdrawal of alcohol.

References

Aragon CMG, Amit Z (1993) Taurine and ethanol induced conditioned taste aversion. Pharmacol Biochem Behav 44: 263–266

Aragon CMG, Trudeau LE, Amit Z (1992) Effect of taurine on ethanol induced changes in open-field locomotor activity. Psychopharmacol 107: 337–340

Beeker KR, Lee RC, Phung HM, Smith CR, Pennington SN (1990) Genetically determined alcohol preference and cyclic AMP binding proteins in mouse brain. Alcohol Clin Exp Res 14: 158–164

Boggan WO, Medberry C, Hopkins DH (1978) Effect of taurine on some pharmacological properties of ethanol. Pharmacol Biochem Behav 9: 469–472

Bowery N (1989) GABAB receptors and their significance in mammalian pharmacology. Trends Pharmacol Sci 10: 401–407

Boyle AE, Smith BR, Amit Z (1992) Microstructural analysis of the effects of THIP, a GABA agonist, on voluntary ethanol intake in laboratory rats. Pharmacol Biochem Behav 43: 1121–1127

Cloninger CR (1987) Neurogenetic adaptative mechanisms in alcoholism. Science 236: 410–416

Daoust M, Saligant C, Lhuintre JP, Moore N, Flipo JC, Boismare F (1987) GABA transmission but not benzodiazepine receptor stimulation, modulates ethanol intake by rats. Alcohol Alcohol 4: 469–472

Deitrich RA, Dunwiddie TV, Harris RA, Erwin VG (1989) Mechanism of action of ethanol initial central nervous system actions. Pharmacol Rev 41: 489–537

Donzanti BA, Yamamoto BK (1988) An improved and rapid HPLC-EC method for the isocaloric separation of amino acids neurotransmitters from brain tissue and microdialysate perfusate. Life Sci 43: 913–922

Gewiss M, Heidbreder C, Opsomer L, Durbin P, De Witte P (1991) Acamprosate and diazepam differentially modulate alcohol-induced behavioural and cortical alterations in rats following chronic inhalation of ethanol vapour. Alcohol Alcohol 26: 129–137

Iida S, Hicki M (1976) Effect of taurine on ethanol-induced sleeping time in mice. J Stud Alcohol 37: 19–26
Kato K, Goto M, Fukuda H (1982) Regulation by divalent cations of ^{3H}baclofen binding to GABAB sites in rat cerebellar membranes. Life Sci 32: 879–887
Kimelberg HK, Cheema M, O'Connor ER, Tong H, Goderie SK, Rossman PA (1993) Ethanol induced aspartate and taurine release from primary astrocyte cultures. J Neurochem 60: 1682–1689
Koob G (1992) Neural mechanisms of drug reinforcement: In: Kalivas PW, Samson HH (eds) The neurobiology of drug and alcohol addiction. New York Academy of Sciences, New York, pp 171–191
Korpi ER (1994) Role of GABAA receptors in the actions of alcohol and in alcoholism: recent advances. Alcohol Alcohol 29, 115–129
Kuriyama K, Ueha T (1992) Functional alterations in cerebral GABAA receptor complex associated with formation of alcohol dependence analysis using GABA-dependent $^{36}Cl^-$ influx into neuronal membrance vesicles. Alcohol Alcohol 27: 335–343
Lhuintre JP, Daoust M, Moore N, Chrétien P, Tran G, Saligaut C, Boismare F, Hillemand B (1985) Ability of calcium bis acetyl homotaurine, a GABA agonist, to prevent relapse in weaned alcoholics. Lancet 1: 1014–1016
Lovinger DM, White G, Weight FF (1989) Ethanol inhibits NMDA-activated ion current in hippocampal neurons. Science 243: 1721–1724
McBride WJ, Chernet E, Dyr W, Lumeng L, Li TK (1993) Densities of Dopamine D (2) receptors are reduced in CNS regions of alcohol-preferring P-rats. Alcohol 10: 387–390
Mehta AK, Ticku MK (1990) Are GABAB receptors involved in the pharmacological effects of ethanol? Eur J Pharmacol 182: 473–480
Murphy JM, McBride WJ, Gatto GJ, Lumeng L, Li TK (1988) Effects of acute ethanol administration on monoamine and metabolic content in forebrain regions of ethanol-tolerant and-nontolerant alcohol preferring (P) rats. Pharmacol Biochem Behav 29: 169–174
Nanima M, Okamoto K, Sakay Y (1982) Taurine acts on presynaptic autoreceptors for GABA in the cerebellum: effects on Ca^{++} influx and GABA release. Jpn J Pharmacol 32: 756–759
Peters TJ, Ward RJ (1988) Role of acetaldehyde in the pathogenesis of alcoholic liver disease. Mol Aspects Medicine 10: 179–190
Rassnick S, D'Amico E, Riley E, Koob GF (1993) GABA antagonist and benzodiazepine partial inverse agonist reduce motivated responding for ethanol. Alcohol Clin Exp Res 17: 480–489
Robinson TE, Whishaw IQ (1988) Normalization of extracellular dopamine in striatum following recovery from a partial unilateral 6-OHDA lesion of the substantia nigra: a microdialysis study in freely moving rats. Brain Res 450: 209–224
Schuller-Levis G, Quinn MR, Wright C, Park E (1994) Taurine protects against oxidant-induced lung injury possible mechanim(s) of action. In: Huxtable RJ, Michalk D (eds) Taurine in health and disease. Plenum, New York, pp 31–39
Smith BR, Robidoux J, Amit Z (1992) GABAergic involvement in the acquistion of voluntary ethanol intake in laboratory rats. Alcohol Alcohol 27: 227–231
Von Wartburg JP, Bühler R (1984) Alcoholism and aldehydism: new biomedical concepts. Lab Invest 50: 5–15
Waller MB, Mcbride WJ, Gatto GL, Lumeng L, Li TK (1984) Intragastric self-infusion of ethanol by ethanol-preferring and -nonpreferring lines of rats. Science 225: 78–80
Watanabe A, Hobara N, Nagashima H (1985) Lowering of liver acetaldehyde but not ethanol concentrations by pretreatment with taurine in ethanol loaded rats. Experientia 41: 1421–1422
Weight FF, Lovinger DM, White G (1991) Alcohol inhibition of NMDA channel function. Alcohol Alcohol [Suppl 1]: 163–169

Event-Related Potentials and EEG as Indicators of Central Neurophysiological Effects of Acamprosate

U. Hegerl, M. Soyka, J. Gallinat, S. Ufer, U. Preuß, R. Bottlender, and H.-J. Möller

Introduction

The homotaurine derivate acamprosate has been proven to be efficient in reducing alcohol intake both in animal models and in human trials. However, the pharmacokinetic and pharmacodynamic properties of this drug in humans and its underlying mechanism of action are not well known. Earlier studies suggested that acamprosate is effective mainly by increasing GABAnergic neurotransmission. More recently the involvement of excitatory amino acid receptors has been discussed. Zeise et al. (1993) found in intracellular in vitro recordings from rat neocortical neurons that the discharge activity evoked by pulses of L-glutamate is reduced by acamprosate. Extracellular in vivo recordings from rat neocortical neurons revealed that excitatory and inhibitory postsynaptic potentials (EPSP, IPSP) as well as responses to locally administered excitatory amino acids [L-glutamate, L-aspartate, L-homocysteate, and *N*-methyl-D-aspartate (NMDA)] are reduced by acamprosate. Serotonergic effects of acamprosate may also be of importance. Acamprosate has been found to increase tryptamine-induced convulsions, to increase serotonin concentrations in both blood and cerebral tissue of rats, and to increase the binding capacity of serotonin 1d and 2 receptors (Nalpas et al. 1990; Daoust et al. 1989).

It is difficult to evaluate the neurochemical effects of acamprosate in humans because no reliable indicators of the various neurochemical systems are available. Event-related potentials (ERP) are of interest in this context. These are cortically generated and depend directly on the spatial and temporal summation of currents induced by EPSP (Mitzdorf 1985, 1994). IPSP probably contribute more indirectly to the generation of the ERP recorded at the scalp. EPSP and IPSP are triggered by the release of excitatory and inhibitory cortical neurotransmitters, and ERP may therefore reflect functional aspects of cortical GABAergic and glutamatergic neurotransmission. In line with this reasoning, an amplitude decrease in auditory ERP was found after administration of MK-801, a NMDA receptor antagonist (Ehlers et al. 1992; Javit et al. 1995), and drugs with GABA-agonistic effects such as benzodiazepines, barbiturates, and ethanol decrease ERP amplitudes (Bond et al. 1974; Pfefferbaum et al. 1980; Frowein et al. 1981; Sinton et al. 1986; Hegerl and Juckel 1993). Because

Psychiatrische Klinik der Ludwig-Maximilians-Universität, 80336 München, Germany acamprosate increases GABAnergic neurotransmission and reduces the function of excitatory amino acid receptors, an amplitude decrease of ERP must be expected.

ERP parameters can reflect not only effects of cortical neurotransmitters but also modulating effects of neuromodulators (e.g., serotonin, acetylcholine) on cortical sensory processing. Such neuromodulators may influence not the amplitude but the more general response pattern of sensory cortices. Converging arguments from preclinical and clinical studies support the hypothesis that the dependence of the auditory evoked N1/P2 amplitude on stimulus intensity (loudness) is correlated inversely with the level of central serotonergic innervation (Hegerl and Juckel 1993; Juckel et al. 1993). In this context dipole source analysis represents an important methodological advance because the N1/P2 subcomponent generated by the primary auditory cortex can be studied at least in part independently from the subcomponent generated by secondary auditory areas. As shown below (Fig. 1), the N1/P2 scalp data can be explained by a tangentially oriented dipole, which reflects activity mainly of the primary auditory cortex, and by a radial dipole, which reflects activity of secondary auditory areas in the lateral temporal cortex. This is important because the serotonergic innervation is high in primary but low in secondary auditory areas (Morrison and Foote 1996; Lewis et al. 1986). Only the intensity dependence of the auditory evoked N1/P2 activity of the tangential dipole has been shown to be promising as an indicator of clinically important aspects of central serotonergic function (Paige et al. 1994; Juckel and Hegerl 1994; Hegerl et al. 1992, 1995a,b) and may therefore reflect serotonergic effects of acamprosate.

We studied the effects of a single dose of acamprosate on ERP in 15 healthy subjects expecting an amplitude decrease in the N1/P2 and P3 components. Because of the serotonergic effects of acamprosate a decrease in intensity dependence of the tangential N1/P2 response of primary auditory cortex also had to be expected. Effects on the resting EEG were also analyzed.

Materials and Methods

Study Design

Effects of acamprosate were investigated within a randomized, double-blind, placebo-controlled study with cross-over design. The time interval between acamprosate or placebo administration was 1 week.

Subjects and Procedure

Fifteen male, healthy, and drug-free volunteers, aged between 21 and 32 years were investigated. The diagnostic process included a physical examination, detailed blood test, drug screening, ECG, and structured interview for the assessment of medical, alcohol, and drug history. Subjects with abnormal findings and a hearing threshold higher than 10 dB were excluded. At 7.30 AM an intravenous permanent catheder was inserted into the subject's nondominant forearm, and electrodes for ERP measurement were fixed. The drug (saline solution or acamprosate, 15 mg/kg) was administered intravenously from 9:15 AM until 9:30. The blinded medication (acamprosate or placebo solutions) was supplied by Lipha. Time "0" was set at 9:30 AM and was used as reference for the flow chart. Resting EEG (3 min with closed eyes) and ERP (N1/P2 and P3 components) were recorded at -60 (8:30 AM), +60 (10:30 AM) and +120 min (11:30 AM). Plasma levels of acamprosate were determined at +60 (10:30) and +120 min (11:30 AM). After transforming acamprosate into a derivative of homotaurine, the quantitative analysis was performed using gas chromatography and mass spectrometry. The analysis was performed by Pharmakin. Pulse rate and blood pressure were measured every 30 min. All subjects were asked about side effects after drug administration and at the end of both study days. A memory test (verbal learning task) was performed, and blood was drawn for endocrinological analysis (data will be reported elsewhere).

AEP Method

Recordings took place in a sound-attenuated and electrically shielded room adjacent to the recording apparatus. The subjects were seated in a slightly reclining chair with a head rest. Evoked responses were recorded using an electrode cap with 29 electrodes. Three additional electrodes were placed (1 nasion, 2 mastoids). Cz was used as reference; Fpz was used as ground. Impedance was below 10 kΩ for each electrode.

N1/P2 Method

During the 17-min recording the subjects were asked to look at a fixation point at the wall in front of them. Sinus tones (1000 Hz, 30 ms duration with 10-ms rise and fall time, ISI randomized between 1800 and 2200 ms) of five intensities (60, 70, 80, 90, 100 dB sound pressure level) were presented binaurally in pseudorandomized form by headphones. The sampling period reached from 200 ms prestimulus to 600 ms poststimulus; 100 sweeps were recorded for each intensity. Before averaging the first five responses to each intensity were excluded in order to reduce short-term habituation effects. Furthermore, for artifact suppression all trials were automatically excluded from averaging when the voltage exceeded ± 50 μV in any of the 32 channels at any point during the averaging period. For each subject the remaining sweeps were averaged separately for the five intensity levels. Dipole source analysis of these potentials was performed using brain electrical source analysis (BESA) with the aim of separating N1/P2 subcomponents overlapping at the scalp. The averaged curves of each subject were entered into BESA, where data reduction, baseline correction, digital filtering (1-20 Hz), and transformation to average reference data took place. To obtain an optimal signal-to-noise ratio for the dipole source analysis a grand average over all intensities, all subjects, and both recording days was calculated. For this data set a basic dipole model was computed for the latency range of the N1/P2 component (66.7–217 ms). The frontopolar (Fp1, Fp2) and the nasion electrodes were not considered in the fit procedure in order to reduce effects of ocular artifacts. Figure 1 presents the resulting basic dipole model. The N1/P2 potentials recorded at the scalp were almost completely explained by one tangential dipole, representing the activity of the primary auditory cortex, and one radial dipole, representing the activity of the secondary auditory cortex in each hemisphere.

To obtain the individual dipole configuration for each subject the sweeps of all intensities and both days of every subject were averaged. The individual dipole model was found by starting with the basic dipole model and adjusting individually the orientation and location of the tangential dipoles. The radial dipoles were not fitted by location or orientation because these explained only a small amount of variance and correspondingly showed higher variability.

The individual curves were calculated according to the individual dipole model. This was established separately for the five stimulus intensities. No additional fitting of location or orientation was performed for the different

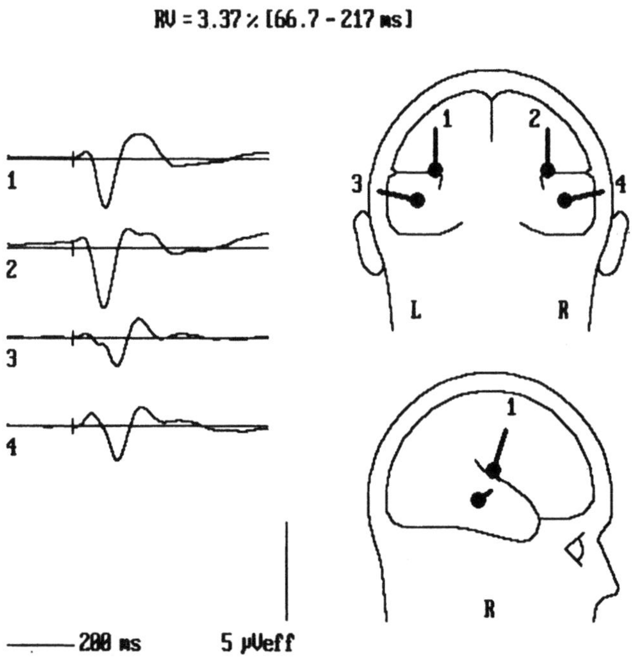

Fig. 1. BESA of grand mean auditory evoked potentials of the 15 healthy subjects. With two tangential (*1, 2*) and two radial dipoles (*3, 4*) 96% of the variance of the scalp potentials in the time range of the N1/P2 component can be explained (*RV*, residual variance). Most of the variance is explained by the dipole source potentials of the tangential dipoles. The dipole source potentials of the radial dipoles are smaller and occur about 40 ms later than those of the tangential dipoles. The tangential dipoles are thought to reflect activity in the superior temporal plane, including primary auditory cortex, and the radial dipoles activity of secondary auditory areas in the lateral temporal cortex

intensities because changes in location or orientation would be confounded with changes in dipole amplitude. The N1/P2 component of the individual dipole source potentials was measured as N1/P2 epoch amplitude in the latency range of 66.7–217 ms. The intensity dependence of the N1/P2 epoch amplitude of the tangential dipole was measured as the median slope. The median slope was calculated from the slopes of all possible straight lines ($n = 10$) connecting the five amplitude values within the amplitude/stimulus intensity function (μVeff/10 dB; Hegerl et al. 1994).

P3 Method

A classical "oddball paradigm" was used. Sinus tones (80 dB) of two frequencies (500 Hz, 80%, 1000 Hz, 20%, ISI 1.5 s) were presented binaurally in pseudorandomized form. The rare 1000 Hz tones did not appear twice consecutively. The sampling period ranged from 200 ms prestimulus to 800 ms poststimulus; 400 sweeps were recorded for the 500 Hz tones, 100 for the 1000 Hz tones. During the stimulation the subjects were asked to keep their eyes closed and to strike a key each time the rare tone appeared. Filtering and averaging were performed as described for the N1/P2 data. The latency and amplitude of the P3 components were determined at Pz and Cz with linked mastoids as reference. The data were digitally filtered between 0.5 and 20 Hz. The P3 component was identified as the most positive peak within 263 and 426 ms. The amplitude was measured in microvolts from the baseline to the peak. Additionally, the P3 component was quantified using the principal components analysis (PCA). For PCA the data were digitally filtered (0.5–20 Hz), and ocular electrodes (Fp1, Fp2, Nz) were excluded. For the remaining 29 electrodes a computing interval between 263 and 426 ms was determined. The most positive amplitude of the main PCA component within the latency range of the P300 was measured.

Resting EEG

The EEG was recorded with Cz as reference (sampling frequency: 256 Hz; low pass: 70 Hz; high pass: 0.16 Hz) and the data were transformed to average reference data. Epochs of 2 s were considered as contaminated with artifacts and were excluded if amplitude values, slope values or curvature values clearly exceeded the normal range (amplitude: 6 times the standard deviation; slope: 9 times the standard deviation; curvature: 12 times the standard deviation). Epochs with amplitudes of more than 100 μV were also excluded. Furthermore, EEGs were inspected visually. Absolute spectral power was calculated for different frequency bands (delta: 1.3–3.5; theta: 3.5–7.5; alpha: 7.5–13; beta: 13–35 Hz) at the leads Oz and Cz. The main frequency in the alpha band was calculated.

Statistics

Effects on acamprosate on N1/P2 amplitudes were analyzed with a three-factor analysis of variance (ANOVA; repeated measurement factor "drug": verum, placebo; repeated measurement factor "time point": 1 h postdrug, 2 h postdrug; repeated measurement factor "intensity": stimulus intensity 60, 70, 80, 90, 100 dB SPL). Effects of acamprosate on the intensity dependence of the tangential dipole N1/P2 amplitudes were analyzed using a two-factor ANOVA (repeated measurement factor "drug": verum, placebo; repeated measurement factor "time point": 1 hour postdrug, 2 h postdrug). Effects of acamprosate on pulse rate and blood pressure were also assessed with a two-factor ANOVA (repeated measurement factor "drug": verum, placebo; repeated measurement factor "time point": 30, 60, 90, 120, 150, 180 min postdrug). The Statistical Package for Social Sciences (SPSS 6.01) was used. All statistical tests were performed in an explorative analysis; therefore the significance levels were not corrected for multiple testing.

Results

The mean plasma concentrations of acetylhomotaurine (in nanograms per milliliter) after slow intravenous infusion were higher after 1 h (27 708 ± 11 997) than after 2 h (12 218 ± 6540) and showed considerable interindividual variability, ranging from 5100 to 51 500 ng/ml. The substance was well tolerated by all subjects. Two subjects reported headache, one on placebo and one on acamprosate. Compared to placebo no significant effects on pulse frequency or systolic or diastolic blood pressure were observed after acamprosate. However, the difference between diastolic and systolic blood pressure tended to increase at about 90 min after acamprosate (interaction effect between the factors "drug" and "time point": $F_{(4;54)}$: 2.45; p=0.057; Fig. 2).

N1/P2 Component

The N1/P2 amplitudes of tangential and radial dipoles (mean amplitude of the five intensity levels) of the pre- and postdrug recordings are presented in Table 1. No significant effects of acamprosate on the amplitude of the N1/P2 component of the radial or tangential dipole activity (interactions between the factors "drug" and "time point") were observed. The N1 component was also analyzed independently; again, no significant effect of acamprosate on the latency or amplitude of this component was found.

Intensity Dependence of the Tangential Dipole N1/P2 Component

The intensity dependence of the tangential dipole N1/P2 activity of the pre- and postdrug recordings are presented in Fig. 3. A significant interaction between the factors "drug" and "time point" was found (F: 9.16; F: 1, 14; p=0.009). The

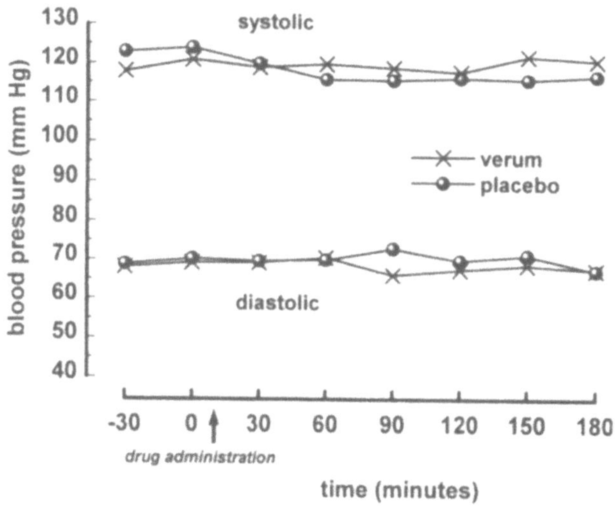

Fig. 2. Systolic and diastolic blood pressure in the placebo and acamprosate session

intensity dependence decreased at the 2-h postdrug recording after acamprosate. When including the predrug values of the intensity dependence in the ANOVA factor "time point," no significant interaction between the factors "drug" and "time point" was found (F: 1.42; F: 2, 28; p=0.258).

P3 Component

In one subject the P3 paradigm was omitted in order to stay within time according to the flow chart. In the remaining 14 subjects no effects of acam-

Table 1. Effects of acamprosate on the N1/P2 amplitude (mean of five intensities) and the P3 amplitude

	Predrug	1 h postdrug	2 h Postdrug
Tangential dipole (N1/P2 epoch ampl.; µV eff)			
Verum	2.07 ± 0.54	2.04 ± 0.51	1.94 ± 0.46
Placebo	2.09 ± 0.57	2.01 ± 0.56	1.87 ± 0.46
Radial dipole (N1/P2 epoch ampl.; µV eff)			
Verum	1.28 ± 0.51	1.34 ± 0.60	1.35 ± 0.65
Placebo	1.40 ± 0.68	1.35 ± 0.66	1.27 ± 0.57
PCA P3 amplitude (nAm)			
Verum	6.57 ± 2.67	6.98 ± 2.98	6.64 ± 2.75
Placebo	6.90 ± 2.40	7.15 ± 2.42	6.67 ± 2.10
P3 amplitude (Pz-linked mastoids; µV)			
Verum	9.80 ± 5.06	10.25 ± 4.90	9.96 ± 4.24
Placebo	10.59 ± 4.33	10.79 ± 4.97	9.90 ± 4.25

All differences between verum and placebo nonsignificant (two-factor ANOVA).

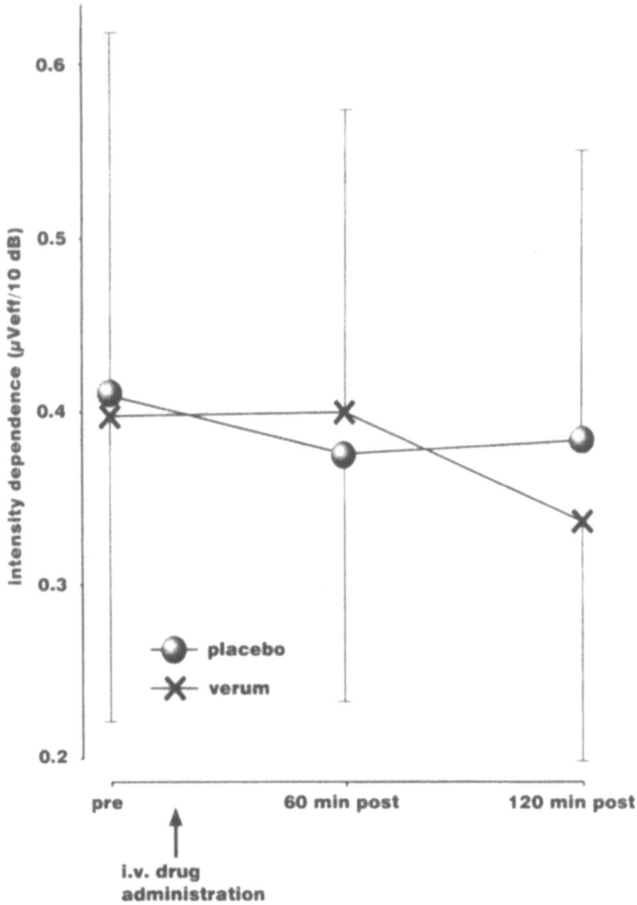

Fig. 3. Intensity dependence of the tangential dipole NI/P2 component (µ V/10 dB) for the pre- and postdrug recordings

prosate on PCA P3 amplitude were detected (Table 1). Analysis of PCA P3 latency and the P3 components measured at Pz and Cz with linked mastoids as reference also revealed no significant acamprosate effects.

Resting EEG

Three subjects had to be excluded because of technical problems with data storage and three others because of insufficient artifact-free resting EEG data. In the remaining nine subjects no effects of acamprosate were detected either on the spectral power values in the different frequency bands or on the main frequencies in the alpha band.

Discussion

The only ERP parameter which tended to be influenced by the acamprosate infusion was the intensity dependence of the tangential N1/P2 dipole activity. The intensity dependence of the tangential dipole activity decreased from the recording 1 h to that 2 h after acamprosate administration. This interaction effect is not very robust, but it is in line with what was expected. There is considerable evidence that intensity dependence of the tangential dipole activity indicates central serotonergic aspects, and that a decrease in this intensity dependence is related to an increase in central serotonergic neurotransmission (Juckel and Hegerl 1994; Hegerl et al. 1992, 1995a,b). Therefore the small effect observed in our study corresponds to reports suggesting serotonin-agonistic effects of acamprosate (Daoust et al. 1989; Nalpas et al. 1990).

However, a single intravenous administration of acamprosate had no significant effects on the other measured neurophysiological parameters. Neither the amplitude nor the latency of the auditory evoked N1/P2 component of tangential or radial dipoles was affected by acamprosate. Furthermore, no effects on P3 amplitude or the spectral power of the resting EEG were detected. This is surprising because a clear effect of acamprosate on EPSP or IPSP discussed in the literature should have been visible in ERP amplitudes. Drugs with GABA-agonistic effects such as benzodiazepines, barbiturates, and ethanol decrease ERP amplitudes (Bond et al. 1974; Pfefferbaum et al. 1980; Frowein et al. 1981; Sinton et al. 1986; Hegerl and Juckel 1993) whereas becuculline, a GABAa receptor antagonist, increases sensory evoked cortical activity (Schroeder et al. 1995). An amplitude decrease in auditory evoked cortical N1 and P2 components as well as hippocampal P3 components was found after administration of MK-801, a NMDA receptor antagonist, in rats (Ehlers et al. 1992). Effects of the same NMDA receptor antagonist on ERP were investigated in monkeys using an oddball paradigm with frequent and deviant auditory stimuli. In this study intravenous administration of MK-801 selectively abolished the difference in negativity (mismatch negativity) elicited by deviant compared to standard stimuli during the latency range of 30–90 ms (Javitt et al. 1995). The lack of P3 amplitude effects of acamprosate in our oddball paradigm argues against strong effects of this drug on NMDA receptor function in our study.

Pharmacokinetic factors may explain the lack of clear effects of acamprosate on ERP and EEG. The plasma levels in our subjects showed a wide range of variation but were clearly higher than those generally observed under steady-state conditions in patients treated with acamprosate. Nevertheless, they may not have been sufficient to achieve pharmacodynamically relevant brain concentrations 2 h after intravenous acamprosate administration. The pharmacokinetic of acamprosate in humans and its behavior in relation to the blood-brain barrier are still not well understood. Acamprosate is thought to cross the blood-brain barrier because of its behavioral effects concerning ethanol consumption and its effects on central neurochemical and neurophysiological functions (Daoust et al. 1992; Gewiss et al. 1991; Rouhani et al. 1986). However, most of these effects have been observed after subacute or chronic treatment with acamprosate or after local cortical administration of acamprosate (Zeise et al. 1993). The finding that acamprosate tends to increase the difference between systolic and diastolic blood pressure could indicate either central or peripheral acamprosate effects. To our knowledge the only study investigating acute effects of acamprosate on evoked potentials is that by Delgrange et al. (1992). In a randomized double-blind study 666 mg acamprosate was administered orally to 12 Patients with alcoholic cirrhosis, and visual evoked P100 latency was determined before and 2 h after drug intake. No significant effects on this parameter was observed.

Therefore it cannot be excluded that the central acamprosate concentrations achieved in our study after a single administration were too low. However, arguments against such a pharmacokinetic explanation of our findings are the observed effects on the intensity dependence of tangential dipole activity and recent results obtained in rats showing a rapid increase in whole-brain and CSF acamprosate levels after both oral and intravenous administration (Durbin et al. 1995).

Another possible explanation of the minimal effects on ERP and EEG parameters in our study is that acamprosate restores ethanol-induced receptor dysfunctions and neurochemical imbalances, and that it develops its neurochemical and neurophysiological effects only in combination with ethanol or during ethanol withdrawal. Some of the reported neurochemical and behavioral effects of acamprosate have been observed in combination with ethanol or in ethanol-dependent animals (Gewiss et al. 1991; Daoust et al. 1992). In a sleep EEG study the main effect of acamprosate was to reverse ethanol-induced sleep EEG changes (Rouhani et al. 1986). Such an interpretation is also supported by the finding that acamprosate seems to counteract the long-lasting changes in latent neuronal hyperexcitability in the withdrawal and postwithdrawal periods (Ziegelgänsberger et al., this volume).

In summary, only the expected decrease in intensity dependence of the tangential dipole N1/P2 component was observable as a tendency 2 h after intravenous administration of acamprosate. This finding supports the postulated serotonin-agonistic effects of acamprosate. In contrast to our expectations, no effects on the other ERP or resting EEG parameter were observed. One explanation for these negative results may be that acamprosate is effective mainly in restoring receptor dysfunctions during withdrawal and postwithdrawal periods and has only minor effects in healthy subjects.

References

Bond AJ, James JC, Lader MH (1974) Physiological and psychological measures in anxious patients. Psychol Med 4: 364–373

Daoust M, Protais P, Boucly P, Tran G, Rinjard P, Dokhan R, Fillion G (1989) Intervention of Aotal on serotoninergic and noradrenergic system. Alcohol Alcohol 24: 370

Daoust M, Legrand E, Gewiss M, Heidbreder C, DeWitte P, Tran G, Durbin P (1992) Acamprosate modulates synaptosomal GABA transmission in chronically alcoholised rats. Pharmacol Biochem Behav 41: 669–674

Delgrange T, Khater J, Capron D, Duron B, Capron JP (1992) Effect of acute administration of acamprosate on the risk of encephalopathy and on arterial pressure in patients with alcoholic cirrhosis. Gastroenterol Clin Biol 16: 687-691
Durbin P, Belleville M, Chabac S (1995) Rat pharmacokinetic profile of acamprosate in plasma, brain and CSF. Poster presented at the ESBRA congress, Stuttgart
Ehlers CL, Kaneko WM, Wall TL, Chaplin RI (1992) Effects of dizocipline (MK-801) and ethanol on the EEG and event-related potentials (EPRs) in rats. Neuropharmacology 31: 369-378
Frowein HW, Gaillard AWK, Varey CA (1981) EP components, visual processing stages and the effect of a barbiturate. Biol Psychol 13: 239-249
Gewiss M, Heidbreder C, Opsomer L, Durbin P, De Witte P (1991) Acamprosate and diazepam differentially modulate alcohol-induced behavioural and cortical alterations in rats following chronic inhalation of ethanol vapour. Alcohol Alcohol 26: 129-137
Hegerl U (1989) Psychopharmaka und kortikale evozierte Potentiale. Fortschr Neurol Psychiatr 57: 267-280
Hegrel U, Juckel G (1993) Intensity dependence of auditory evoked potentials as indicator of central serotonergic neurotransmission - a new hypothesis. Biol Psychiatry 33: 173-187
Hegerl U, Wulff H, Müller-Oerlinghausen B (1992) Intensity dependence of auditory evoked potentials and clinical response to prophylactic lithium medication: a replication study. Psychiatry Res 44: 181-191
Hegerl U, Gallinat J, Mrowinski D (1994) Intensity dependence of auditory evoked dipole source activity. Int J Psychophysiol 17: 1-13
Hegerl U, Lipperheide K, Juckel G, Schmidt LG, Rommelspacher H (1995a) Antisocial tendencies and cortical sensory evoked responses in alcoholism. Alcohol Clin Exp Res 19: 31-36
Hegerl U, Gallinat J, Mrowinksi D (1995b) Sensory cortical processing and the biological basis of personality. Biol Psychiatry 37: 467-472
Javitt DC, Schroeder CE, Steinschneider M, Arezzo JC, Ritter W, Vaughan HG (1995) Cognitive event-related potentials in human and non-human primates: implication for the PCP/NMDA model of schiziohrenia. In: Karmos G, Molnár M, Csépe V, Czigler I, Desmedt EJ (eds) Perspectives of event-related potentials research (EEG suppl 44). Elsevier, Amsterdam, pp 161-175
Juckel G, Hegerl U (1994) Evoked potentials, serotonin, and suicidality. Pharmacopsychiatry 27: 27-29
Juckel G, Molnár M, Hegerl U, Csépe V, Karmos G (1993) Intensity dependence of auditory evoked potentials as indicator of central serotonergic neurotransmission - first evidence in the behaving cat. Pharmacopsychiatry 26: 166
Lewis DA, Campbell MJ, Foote SL, Morrison JH (1986) The monoaminergic innervation of primate neocortex. Hum Neurobiol 5: 181-188
Mitzdorf U (1985) Current source-density method and application in cat cerebral cortex: investigation of evoked potentials and EEG phenomena. Physiol Rev 65: 37-91
Mitzdorf U (1994) Properties of cortical generators of event-related potentials. Pharmacopsychiatry 27: 49-51
Morrison JH, Foote SL (1986) Noradrenergic and serotoninergic innervation of cortical, thalamic, and tectal visual structures in old and new world monkeys. J Comp Neurol 243: 117-138
Nalpas B, Dabadie H, Parot P, Paccalin J (1990) L'acamprosate: de la pharmacologie à la clinique. Encephale 16: 175-179
Paige SR, Fitzpatrick DF, Kline JP, Balogh SE, Hendricks SE (1994) Event-related potential amplitude/intensity slopes predict response to antidepressants. Neuropsychobiology 30: 197-201
Pfefferbaum A, Horvath TB, Roth WT et al (1980) Acute and chronic effects of ethanol on event related potentials. In: Begleiter H (ed) Biological effects of alcohol. Plenum, New York, pp 625-640
Rouhani S, Tran G, Lepaideur F, Durlach J, Poenaru S (1986) Etudes electropolygraphiques (EPG) des effets aigus de l'ethanol (ETOH) sur le sommeil chez des adultes volontaires sains recevant de l'acetyl-homotaurinate de calcium (Aota Ca). Bull Soc Fr Alcool 4: 59-62
Schroeder CE, Steinschneider M, Javitt DC, Tenke CE, Givre SJ, Mehta AD, Simpson GV, Arezzo JC, Vaughan HG (1991) Localisation of ERP generators and identification of underlying neural processes. In: Karmos G, Molnár M, Csépe V, Czigler I, Desmedt EJ (eds) Perspectives of event-related potentials research (EEG suppl 44). Elsevier, Amsterdam, pp 55-75

Sinton C, McCullough J, Ilmoniemi R, Etienne P (1986) Modulation of a auditory evoked magnetic fields by benzodiazepines. Neuropsychobiology 16: 215–218

Zeise ML, Kasparov S, Capogna M, Ziegelgänberger W (1993) Acamprosate (calciumacethyhomotaurinate) decreases postsynaptic potentials in the rat neocortex: possible involvement of excitatory amino acid receptors. Eur J Pharmacol 231: 47–52

Effects of Acamprosate on Verbal Learning in Healthy Young Subjects

N. Kathmann, M. Soyka, J. Gallinat, and U. Hegerl

Introduction

Several studies have shown acamprosate to increase abstinence rates in weaned alcoholics compared to placebo. This makes the substance a promising "anticraving" drug of high clinical importance (Paille et al. 1995; Soyka, this volume; H. Sass, M. Soyka, K. Mann, W. Zieglgänsberger 1995, Relapse Prevention by Acamprosate: Results from a Placebo Controlled Study in Alcohol Dependence, in press).

The suggested mechanisms of action of acamprosate include an antagonistic effect on the postsynaptic efficacy of excitatory amino-acids (L-glutamate and others) resulting in a lower neuronal excitability (Zeise et al. 1993; Zieglgänsberger, this volume). Glutamate plays an important role in memory processes as the *N*-methyl-D-aspartate (NMDA) receptors are involved in hippocampal long-term potentiation (LTP). LTP is an acknowledged model of memory formation and neuronal plasticity at a cellular level (Collingridge and Bliss 1987; McEntee and Crook 1993). Decreased glutamatergic activity may impair learning and memory formation via reduced LTP, as suggested by research in animals (Morris et al. 1986; McEntee and Crook 1993). On the other hand, excitatory neurotransmitters have neurotoxic effects under certain conditions, for example, by inducing influx of Ca_{2+} into the cell. Thus, reducing the effects of excitatory amino acids may offer a strategy to prevent neuronal degeneration to some degree (Lawlor and Davis 1992). For these reasons it can be speculated that acamprosate affects learning and memory due to its dampening effects on excitatory neurotransmission.

Although few adverse side effects have been reported in clinical studies with acamprosate, the possible impairment of learning and memory formation caused by this drug has not yet been sufficiently addressed. The present experimental study investigated the short-term effects of a single administration of acamprosate in healthy volunteers using a standardized verbal learning task.

Psychiatrische Klinik der Ludwig-Maximilians-Universität, Nußbaumstr. 7, 80336 München, Germany

Material and Methods

Subjects

The subjects in this study were 15 healthy right-handed male subjects between 21 and 32 years. They were paid for participation and gave written, informed consent to the study. Subjects were screened by a physical examination and blood laboratory tests to be free of relevant medical or psychiatric disease. Subjects taking medication for therapeutic reasons or abusing drugs and/or alcohol were not included.

Procedure

The study was carried out using a double-blind, two-period, cross-over design with a 1-week interval between periods. Subjects were randomized into one of two groups. Group 1 received placebo in the first experimental session and 15 mg/kg acamprosate in the second session; group 2 received the substances in the reversed order. The blinded solutions were supplied by Lipha. Subjects arrived in the ward at 7:30 A.M. An intravenous permanent catheter was inserted in the subject's nondominant forearm, and electrodes for EEG measurement were fixed. The drug (saline solution or acamprosate) was administered intravenously at 9:15 over 15 min. Pulse rate and blood pressure were recorded every 30 min from 9:00 until 12:00 A.M. Acamprosate blood levels were determined at 10:30 and 11:30 A.M. Between 8:30 and 12:00 A.M. a set of EEG and event-related potential recordings were conducted (see Hegerl et al., this volume). The verbal learning task was performed at 9:00 (immediately prior to drug application) and at 11:15 A.M.

Task

The verbal learning task allows assessment of the acquisition of new verbal information and of the retrieval from short-term memory (Warburton and Rusted 1989). In addition, the course of learning across repeated trials can be evaluated. There were four such learning trials in succession within each task. The experimenter read aloud the words of the list to the subject at a rate of one word every 2 s. The subject was then requested immediately to recall the words. The maximum time allowed for reproducing the words was 90 s. The procedure of hearing the words and subsequently recalling them was repeated another two times in identical manner with the same list. The fourth trial included a distraction task after hearing the words. Subjects were to count aloud backwards in steps of seven beginning from 200. A delayed recall test was then given to measure memory consolidation. The experimenter noted the words produced by the subject and made records of correctly recalled words and intrusions after each learning trial. As the whole task was given four times (before and after placebo, before and after acamprosate) there were four different lists of words to avoid practice effects across tasks. The order of the lists was randomized among subjects. The lists were matched for imagery, concreteness, meaningfulness, and frequency of the words (Baschek et al. 1977).

Statistical Analyses

A memory performance score was computed for each learning trial by subtracting the number of intrusions from the number of correctly recalled items. These scores were analyzed by repeated measures analysis of variance (ANOVA). The order of drugs was included as a between-subjects factor. Period (sessions 1 and 2), time (pre-and postdrug), and learning trials (1–4) were the within-subject factors. The effect of drug was tested by the interaction of order by period of time. When the four level factor learning was involved, error probabilities were corrected with Greenhouse-Geisser's ε.

Results

The means and standard errors of means of the memory scores are shown in Fig. 1. Performance increased from trial 1 to trial 3 and remained almost stable in trial 4. The results of the four-factorial ANOVA indicated that order of drugs did not affect learning and memory performance ($F_{(1,13)}=0.15$; ns). This means that the effects of drug administration did not carry over. Also, the main effect of periods was not significant ($F_{(1,13)}=1.20$; ns). No change from pre to post-drug measures was found across drugs and trials ($F_{(1,13)}=2.05$; ns). Learning across repeated trials within sessions was statistically highly significant ($F_{(3,39)}=148.30$; $p < 0.001$). The drug effect was confirmed statistically by the significant interaction of order by period of time ($F_{(1,13)} = 6.62$; $p < 0.05$). Figure 1 shows that there was a decrease in memory performance from pre- to postdrug

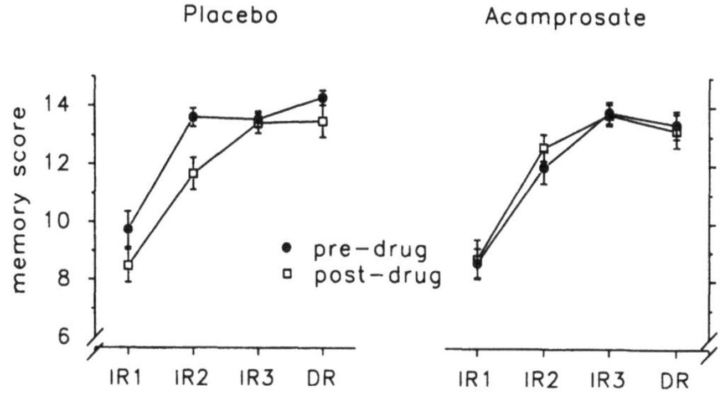

Fig. 1. Means ± SEM of the memory scores (correctly recalled words minus intrusions) for the four learning trials, recorded before (-15 min) and after (+120 min) drug administration under placebo and acamprosate conditions. *IR 1–3*, Immediate recall trials 1–3; *DR*, delayed recall trial 4

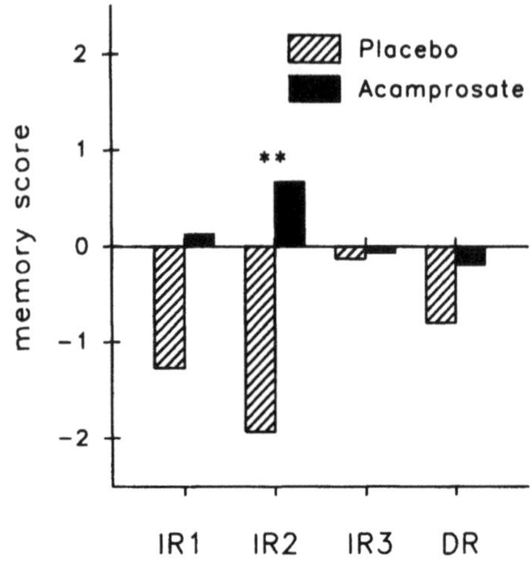

Fig. 2. Changes of memory scores from pre-to postdrug recordings for the four learning trials under placebo and acamprosate. *IR 1–3*, Immediate recall trials 1–3; *DR*, delayed recall trial 4. ** $p < 0.01$ (paired *t*-test)

measures under placebo that was not seen under acamprosate. In addition, a tendency was found for this effect to vary with learning trials ($F_{(3,39)}$.= 2.50; $p < 0.10$). To express the drug effect more directly, change scores (before vs. after) were computed separately for the two drug conditions and each of the learning trials. Figure 2 shows these change scores. To better specify the drug effect, separate paired *t* tests were computed comparing placebo and acamprosate during each of the four learning trials. Only after the second presentation of the words was the difference between drugs significant (t=3.63; $p < 0.01$). In a further 2 (drugs) × 2 (learning trials 1 and 2) ANOVA, computed with the change values, it was tested whether the slope of newly acquired words was changed by acamprosate. The interaction of drug by learning trial ($F_{(1,14)}$ = 1.47; ns) was not significant, thus confirming the lack of such a difference. Memory consolidation was suggested to be reflected in changes of performance scores from trial 3 (immediate recall) to trial 4 (delayed recall). However, there was no significant interaction of drug by trials ($F_{(1,14)}$ = 0.42; ns). Therefore the hypothesis of differential memory consolidation due to placebo or acamprosate administration must be rejected.

Discussion

In the present experiment no detrimental effect of acamprosate on memory functions could be observed. With the proposed mechanism of action of acamprosate as a NMDA antagonist, an impairment of both acquisitions and recall of material to be learned was expected from animal experiments using NMDA receptor antagonists such as phencyclidine or dizocilpine (MK-801; Handelmann et al. 1987; Wozniak et al. 1990; McLamb et al. 1990). Immediate recall of the learned words was tested after each of three learning trials, and performance was not worse under acamprosate on any occasion. Also, the slope of the learning curve did not distinguish between drug conditions. Thus, working memory seemed to be unaffected by the experimental treatment. Secondary (or long-term) memory, which requires consolidation of working memory contents, was measured by the recall performance after a distraction task. Diminished LTP induced by the hypothesized glutamate-antagonistic effect of acamprosate should most likely produce deficits in memory consolidation and consequently lower the number of recalled items from long-term memory learned under acamprosate. However, we found no such deficit with the task used here. It should also be noted that the data on evoked potentials revealed no marked effects of acamprosate indicating a reduced neuronal excitability (Hegerl et al., this volume). In animal studies the amplitudes of evoked potentials decreased after the administration of MK-801, a glutamate receptor antagonist (Ehlers et al. 1992). Our negative results lend no support to the hypothesis that acamprosate acts as a NMDA antagonist. However, at least with regard to the verbal learning data, this conclusion might be premature. The time window that we used for recording memory effects may have been too narrow to monitor these completely. Blood levels of acamprosate were falling even at the time of memory measurement. Some other limitations of the study are discussed in greater detail by Hegerl et al. (this volume). Nevertheless, the only statistically significant effect of acamprosate in the memory study was against our expectation and showed an *improvement* in recall performance after the second learning trial. Certainly, this effect is too selective to be substantial, and it is difficult to explain on the basis of the suggested mechanisms of action of this drug.

In addition to considering the neurophysiological aspects of acamprosate, it is important to evaluate the results from a clinical perspective. Previous experience with the use of acamprosate in alcoholic patients has revealed only few side effects. Complaints regarding cognitive deficits, especially memory impairment, have not been reported so far. The present experimental study supports the impression from less controlled observations that acamprosate shows no detrimental effects on memory. However, further experimental studies with patients treated during an adequately long period (i.e., at least several weeks) should be conducted to confirm this under everyday clinical conditions.

References

Baschek I-L, Bredenkamp J, Oehrle B, Wippich W (1977) Bestimmung der Bildhaftigkeit (I), Konkretheit (C) und der Bedeutungshaltigkeit (m') von 800 Substantiven. Z Exp Ang Psychol 24: 353–396

Collingridge GL, Bliss TVP (1987) NMDA receptors – their role in long-term potentiation. Trends Neurosci 10: 288–293

Ehlers CL, Kaneko WM, Wall TL, Chaplin RI (1992) Effects of dizocilpine (MK-801) and ethanol on the EEG and event-related potentials (ERPs) in rats. Neuropharmacology 31: 369–378

Handelmann GE, Contreras PC, O'Donohue TL (1987) Selective memory impairment by phencyclidine in rats. Eur J Pharmacol 140: 69–73

Lawlor BA, Davis KL (1992) Does modulation of glutamatergic function represent a viable therapeutic strategy in Alzheimer's disease? Biol Psychiatry 31: 337–350

McEntee WJ, Crook TH (1993) Glutamate: its role in learning, memory, and the aging brain. Psychopharmacology 111: 391–401

McLamb RL, Williams LR, Nanry KP, Wilson WA, Tilson HA (1990) MK-801 impedes the acquisition of a spatial memory task in rats. Pharmacol Biochem Behav 37: 41–45

Morris RGM, Anderson E, Lynch GS, Baudry M (1986) Selective impairment of learning and blockade of long-term potentiation of an N-methyl-D-aspartate receptor antagonist, AP5. Nature 319: 774–776

Paille FM, Guelfi JD, Perkins AC, Royer RJ, Steru L, Parot P (1995) Double-blind randomized multicenter trial of acamprosate in maintaining abstinence from alcohol. Alcohol Alcohol 30: 239–247

Warburton DM, Rusted JM (1989) Memory assessment. In: Hindmarch I, Stonier PD (eds) Human psychopharmacology: measures and methods, vol 2 Wiley, New York, pp 155–178

Wozniak DF, Olney JW, Kettinger L III, Price M, Miller JP (1990) Behavioral effects of MK-801 in the rat. Psychopharmacology 101: 47–56

Zeise ML, Kasparow S, Capogna M, Zieglgänsberger W (1993) Acamprosate (calciumhomotaurinate) decrease postsynaptic potentials in the rat neocortex: possible involvement of excitatory amino acid receptors. Eur J Pharmacol 231: 47–52

Acamprosate in Clinical Practice: The French Experience

H.-J. Aubin

Introduction

Acamprosate is an adjunct for the treatment of alcohol dependence due to its anticraving and relapse-reducing properties. It was developed by French pharmaceutic industry and has been marketed in this country since 1989. Since then, acamprosate has been prescribed over 2 million times by French practitioners to patients suffering from alcohol abuse or dependence. In addition, seven clinical trials have collected data on 2824 patients and have confirmed its efficacy and good tolerance. Ten other clinical studies, including 2695 patients, have recently been conducted in Europe. The methodological issues and results of these European studies are the subjects of separate chapters in this volume (A.S. Potgieter, and P. Lehert). The aim of this chapter is to synthesize French clinical experience with acamprosate.

The French Sociocultural Context

Europe has the highest per capita alcohol consumption in the world. In 1990 this exceeded 8 l of pure alcohol in 15 of the 26 WHO member states for which data are available (WHO 1993). Among these countries France has the highest declared alcohol consumption: 11.9 l per capita in 1991 (Association Nationale de Prévention de l'Alcoolisme 1993). It is noteworthy, however, that both alcohol consumption and deaths from cirrhosis of the liver are rapidly decreasing in France (24% and 42%, respectively, between 1970 and 1988; WHO 1993). The decrease in alcohol consumption is due essentially to the decrease in daily wine intake (Association Nationale de Prévention de l' Alcoolisme 1993). However, wine remains by far the most consumed alcoholic beverage, accounting for 64.3% of alcohol intake (Haut Comité de la Santé Publique 1995). Spirits, beer, and cider account, respectively, for 20.3%, 14.3%, and 1.1% of alcohol intake.

There is a complete lack of well-structured epidemiological surveys on alcohol abuse and dependence prevalence in the general population in France. The only information on the general population is an indirect figure on the

Centre d'Alcoologie, Hôpital Emile Roux, 94456 Limeil-Brévannes Cedex, France prevalence of alcohol dependence based on the incidence of mortality from cirrhosis of the liver; the prevalence of alcohol dependence was in 1989 estimated at 5% among adults aged over 18 years (Haut Comité de la Santé Publique 1995). Telephone surveys showed that the prevalence of excessive drinkers (four or more per day in men and three drinks or more per day in women) was 18.6% in the French general population over age 15: 28.1% in men and 9.8% in women. Although life-styles are changing in France, drinking is still essentially of the Mediterranean type. The traditional drinking pattern is typically wine during meals, preceded by aperitif, and on an everyday basis. Drinking among the young has been approximating that in northern Europe: binge drinking of spirits or beer on weekends. Peer pressure to drink is common in family, friendship, and professional circles.

The management of alcohol dependence in France is divided between:

- Abstinence, as the unquestioned therapeutic mean, shared by many addiction professionals, in particular at the Société Française d'Alcoologie, and self-help organizations. These professionals ban controlled drinking, as this goal cannot be achieved on a long-term basis.
- Reduction in consumption or alcohol-related harm, shared by some less informed public health professionals and general practitioners. Some well-informed addiction physicians sometimes advocate controlled drinking. However, they usually advocate this option less publicly.

It is notable that there is often confusion between the therapeutic goal, for example, the enhancement of life quality, and the principal therapeutic mean, which is usually abstinence. In this context, it was unlikely that a medication would be developed to reduce alcohol consumption or alcohol-related harm in alcoholics, and therefore acamprosate development, from preclinical findings indicating alcohol intake reduction in animals (Boismare et al. 1984; Le Magnen et al. 1987b), focused on relapse prevention in humans.

Efficacy Trials

The first clinical study (Lhuintre et al. 1985) was a randomized double-blind, placebo-controlled single-center trial on 85 alcoholic patients. Inclusion criteria were: daily alcohol intake above 200 g/day, alcohol dependence indicated by the morning withdrawal syndrome or at least two failed attempts at weaning by medical methods or self-help groups, elevated γ-glutamyltranspeptidase (GGT) and mean corpuscular volume (MCV). No concomitant relapse prevention therapies (apomorphine, disulfiram, self-help groups) were allowed. The only concomitant treatment allowed was meprobamate and vitamins B_1 and B_6. Patients were treated with 25 mg/kg acamprosate daily or placebo during the 3 months of follow-up after their hospital discharge. At the end of the trial 61% of the patients did not relapse in the acamprosate group vs. 32% in the placebo group ($p<0.02$). Patients successfully treated by acamprosate reported a decreased interest in alcohol.

This positive clinical result led to a further randomized double-blind, placebo-controlled multicenter trial (Lhuintre et al. 1990) on 569 alcoholic patients. Inclusion criteria were: alcohol dependence indicated by the morning withdrawal syndrome or at least two failed attempts at durable detoxification or organization of the patient's life-style to prevent any break in the alcohol supply, elevated GGT and MCV. Concomitant treatment with sedative drugs was permitted throughout the trial. Treatment (acamprosate at 1.33 g/day or placebo) was started on the day of hospital discharge (5–30 days after admission). Follow-up and treatment lasted 3 months. The major finding of this study was a significant difference in GGT level at the end of the study, in favor of acamprosate (Fig. 1). Clinical signs of physical dependence were also significantly less frequent in acamprosate group. In addition, a number of statistical trends favored Acamprosate: anxiety, transaminase, and global therapeutic effect assessed by the physician and by the patient.

Based on the results of these studies acamprosate was marketed in France in 1989 for the indication of alcoholism, with the recommended dose of 1.33 g/day (four tablets) and recommended duration of 3 months. Subsequent phase 4 clinical studies confirmed acamprosate efficacy.

An open trial was performed in a military occupational health institution (Dubourg et al. 1990) on 77 patients hospitalized for alcohol detoxification. No patient was lost to follow-up in this setting. Patients received acamprosate (1.33 g/day if under 60 kg bodyweight and 2 g/day if over 60 kg) at discharge. Continuous abstinence rates were 61% and 40.2% at 6 and 12 months' follow-up, respectively.

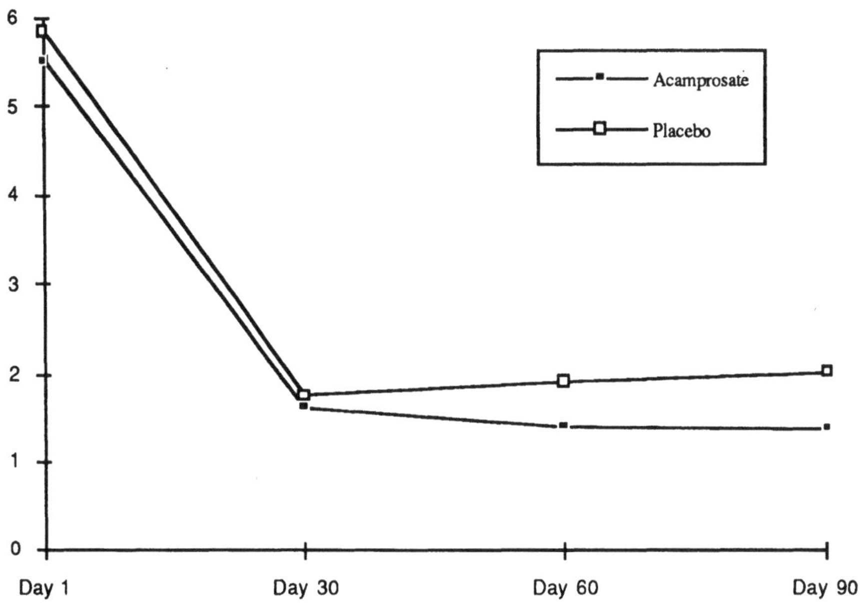

Fig. 1. GGT level (times normal) at different assessments. At days 60 and 90: $p<0.05$. (From Lhuintre et al. 1990)

Another noncomparative, multicenter open trial included 860 patients with the diagnosis of alcohol abuse or dependence [criteria of the *Diagnostic and Statistical Manual of Mental Disorders*, 3rd revised edition (DSM III-R); Ades et al. 1992). Patients were treated with 1.33 g/day acamprosate during the 3 months' follow-up, time after which 71% of the completers and 53% of those with intention to treat were abstinent. Of the nonabstinent patients at 3 months' follow-up, 64% were rated by the investigator as having a moderate alcohol intake.

Pelc et al. (1992) published the results of a multicenter double-blind, parallel, placebo-controlled trial on 102 alcohol-dependent patients (DSM III-R criteria), with a 6 months' follow-up. Acamprosate had a significant effect on abstinence rates at each follow-up assessment (from day 30 to day 180), mean number of days without alcohol, global clinical impression scale, and compliance with treatment (excess of drop-outs in the placebo group).

Finally, the results of a large multicenter double-blind, parallel, placebo-controlled trial have recently been published (Paille et al. 1995). After detoxification each of the 538 alcohol-dependent patients included (DSM III-R criteria) was randomly assigned to placebo, acamprosate at 1.33 g/day, or acamprosate at 2 g/day. Trial medication was started 7–28 days after the last drink. Concomitant prescription of the antidepressant maprotiline and the anxiolytic lorazepam was permitted. Treatment lasted 12 months and was followed by a single-blind 6-month period on placebo. Globally the results show a dose effect in favor of acamprosate at 2 g/day. At all assessment points the percentage of patients continuously abstinent was highest in the high-dose acamprosate group and lowest in the placebo group, with intermediate values for the low-dose Acamprosate group. The overall difference was significant at 6 months' ($p<0.02$) but not at 12 months' follow-up ($p=0.096$). Analysis of abstinence since the last assessment at each visit showed that abstinence rates in the acamprosate groups were always significantly superior to those for placebo except at 3 months' follow-up (Fig. 2).

This difference persisted at 18 months' follow-up, although all patients had been treated with placebo since the 12 months' follow-up visit. Time to first relapse was significantly longer in the high-dose acamprosate group compared to the placebo group (153 ± 197 days versus 102 ± 165 days, $p=0.005$), the low-dose acamprosate figure lying between these (135 ± 189 days). The cumulative period of abstinence (defined as the total number of days of abstinence, whether continuous or not) was also longer in the high-dose acamprosate group compared to the placebo group (223 ± 134 days versus 173 ± 126 days, $p=0.005$), low-dose acamprosate again lying between these (198 ± 133 days). Acamprosate thus appears to induce a dose-dependent improvement in the duration of patients' follow-up (Fig. 3).

At 12 months' follow-up 54.9% of patients remained in the trial in the high-dose acamprosate group, 47.3% in the low-dose acamprosate group, and 35.6% in the placebo group ($p=0.006$). A significant difference between groups persisted after the 18 months' post-treatment period. Patients' craving for alcohol was assessed at the major visits by the investigator on a three-point ordinal scale. The only significant group difference was at the 3 months' follow-up,

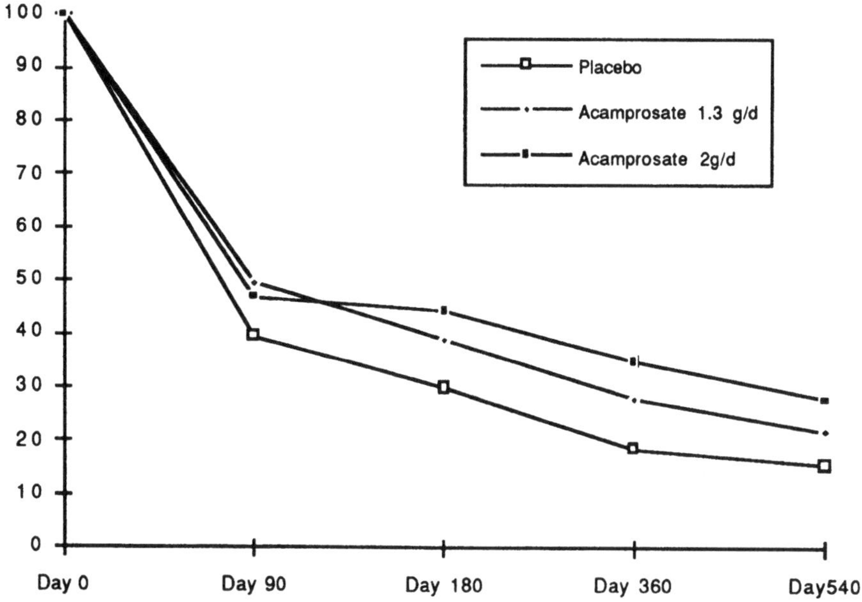

Fig. 2. Percentage of patients abstinent at each assessment. At day 180: $p<0.001$; at day 360: $p<0.001$; at day 540: $=0.002$. (From Paille et al. 1995)

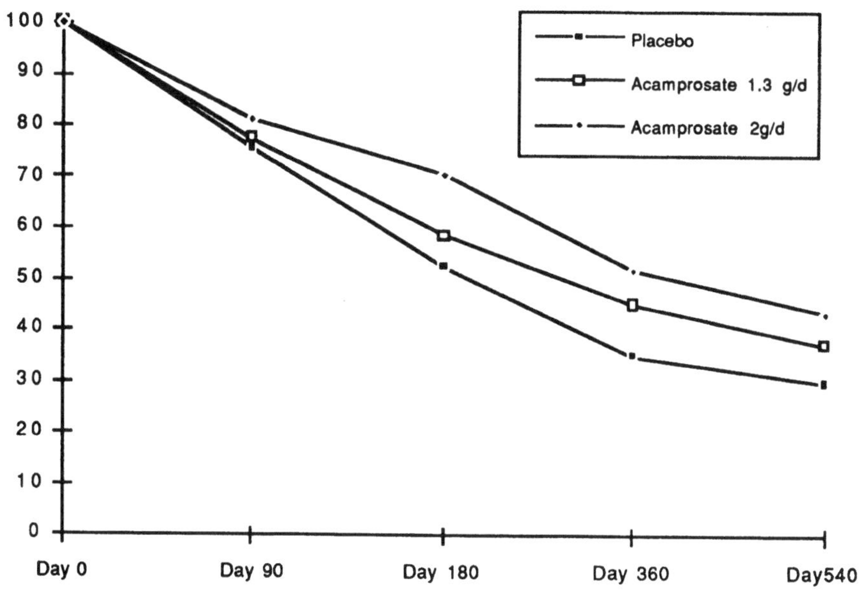

Fig. 3. Percentage of patients remaining in the trial at different assessments. At day 180: $p=0.002$; at day 360: $p=0.005$; at day 540: $p=0.034$. (From Paille et al. 1995)

when 59.4% of the patients in the high-dose acamprosate group compared with 40% in the placebo group reported no craving, GGT assessments confirmed clinical results: the percentage of patients with a GGT level within the normal range was significantly higher with acamprosate than with placebo at 6 months' and at 12 months' follow-up.

These phase 4 data led to modification of the marketing conditions in France: the recommended daily dose is now 2 g and the recommended duration of treatment is 1 year.

Tolerance

The good tolerance of acamprosate has been confirmed by the various double-blind and open efficacy trials reported above, by a specific tolerance trial (Aubin et al. 1995), and by postmarketing surveillance.

On the whole, acamprosate causes no serious adverse event. The most common side effect is soft stools or diarrhea, which was dose-dependent in the study published by Paille et al. (1995). The only other side effect that appears significantly more frequently with acamprosate than with placebo in controlled trials is vertigo (p=0.05; Lhuintre et al. 1990). Preclinical data show that acamprosate has no interaction with ethanol (Le Magnen et al. 1987a). This has been largely confirmed by everyday practice and postmarketing surveillance. Moreover, acamprosate reduces the alcohol withdrawal syndrome in rats (Gutierrez et al. 1987). No pharmacological interaction between acamprosate and other medications has been observed in efficacy trials or postmarketing surveillance. An open tolerance trial addressed specifically this issue (Aubin et al. 1995). This study examined the safety of combining acamprosate, as soon as the patient had been weaned from alcohol, with the drugs usually prescribed to prevent the alcohol withdrawal syndrome. It was an open controlled multicenter trial on parallel groups for a period of 15 days and included 591 alcohol-dependent (DSM III) patients admitted to hospital for alcohol detoxification. There were four treatment groups. All the patients were given acamprosate (2 g/day) and vitamins B_1 and B_6. The patients in group A were also given tetrabamate, those in group B meprobamate, and those in group C oxazepam; the patients in group D received no drug to prevent withdrawal symptoms. Tolerability of the treatment was evaluated in a repeated fashion by registering of spontaneous complaints, a systematic questionnaire concerning complaints, revised clinical institute withdrawal assessment for alcohol (CIWA-Ar) scale, a craving for alcohol scale and a laboratory investigation. The adverse events were defined by means of analysis of imputation of the complaints to the treatment. The results showed that the tolerability (in terms of adverse events, withdrawal syndrome, and craving for alcohol) of the combination of acamprosate and vitamins B_1 and B_6 was unchanged or improved by adding tetrabamate, meprobamate, or oxazepam (Figs. 4–6).

Acamprosate may therefore be used concomitantly with alcohol detoxification in combination with drugs usually prescribed to prevent the withdrawal syndrome, starting with the beginning of alcohol detoxification.

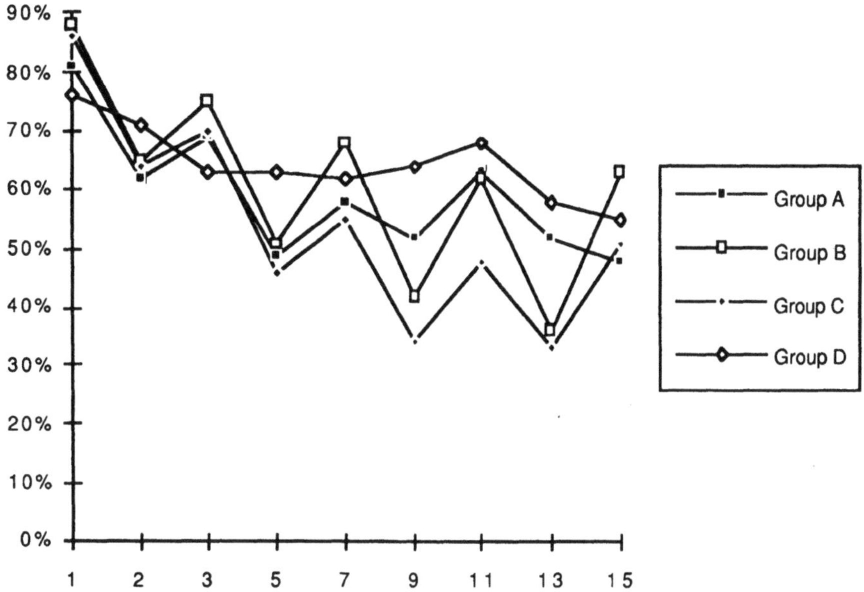

Fig. 4. Percentage of patients complaining of at least one adverse event (even if minimal) at each assessment (from day 1 to day 15). *Group A*, acamprosate + tetrabamate, *group B*, acamprosate + meprobamate; *group C*, acamprosate + oxazepam; *group D*, acamprosate alone. (From Aubin et al. 1995)

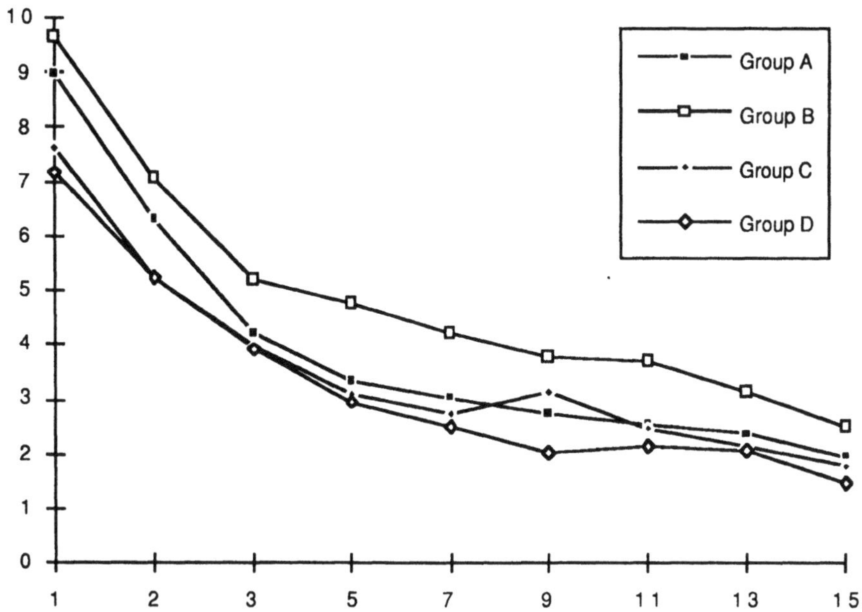

Fig. 5. Mean CIWA-Ar score at each assessment (from day 1 to day 15). *Group A*, acamprosate + tetrabamate; *group B*, acamprosate + meprobamate; *group C*, acamprosate + oxazepam; *group D*, acamprosate alone. (From Aubin et al. 1995)

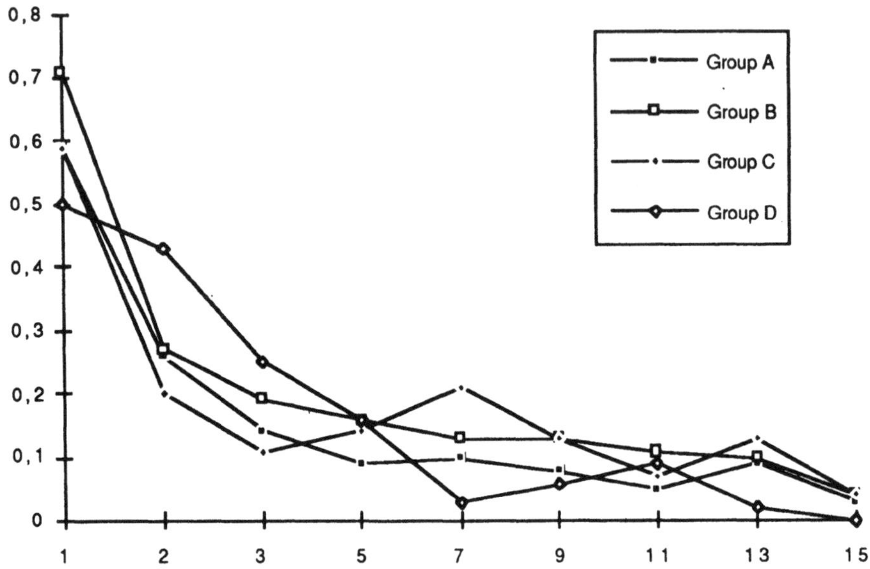

Fig. 6. Mean craving score at each assessment (from day 1 to day 15). *Group A*, acamprosate + tetrabamate; *group B*, acamprosate + meprobamate; *group C*, acamprosate + oxazepam; *group D*, acamprosate alone. (From Aubin et al. 1995)

Conclusion

Acamprosate has shown its efficacy as an adjunct in the treatment of alcohol dependence. Its main effects are:

- Prevention of relapse, assessed by an effect on abstinence rates in the medium-term and long-term (up to 18 months), time to first relapse, and cumulative period of abstinence
- Improvement in patients' clinic attendance, with lower drop-out rates in patients treated with Acamprosate than with placebo
- Possible reduction in alcohol craving

The efficacy of acamprosate is supported by the dose effect found in the study of Paille et al. (1995). Acamprosate has a good tolerance profile: (a) no major adverse effect, (b) no pharmacodependence, and (c) no interaction with ethanol or current medications. Acamprosate has been prescribed by French physicians over 2 million times since its initial marketing in 1989. French experience with this drug is obviously positive, since the prescription rate continues to grow. It has now become a standard element of alcohol relapse prevention strategy, along with all other medical, behavioral, psychological, social, and self-help components.

References

Ades J, Granger B, Parot P (1992) Intérêt d'Aotal chez le malade alcoolique en pratique médicale courante. Essai multicentrique sur 860 patients. Inf Psy 5: 517-521

Association Nationale de Prévention de l'Alcoolisme (1993) Statistiques - edition 1993. Association Nationale de Prévention de l'Alcoolisme, Paris

Aubin HJ, Lehert P, Beaupere B, Parot P, Barrucand D (1995) Tolerability of the combination of acamprosate with drugs used to prevent alcohol withdrawal syndrome. Alcoholism 31: 25-38

Boismare F, Daoust M, Moore N, Saligaut C, Lhuintre JP, Chretien P, Durlach J (1984) A homotaurine derivative reduces the voluntary intake of ethanol by rats: are cerebral GABA receptors involved? Pharmacol Biochem Behav 21: 787-789

Dubourg C, Favre JD, Parot P (1990) Essai thérapeutique contrôlé de l'acamprosate dans le maintien du sevrage alcoolique pendant une année au sein d'une structure multicentrique de médecine du travail. Résultats dfinitifs à J 90 et partiels à J 180. Alcoologie 12: 96-103

Gutierrez S, Daoust M, Rinjard P, Lhuintre JP, Boismare F (1987) L'acétylhomotaurinate de calcium, molécule à propriétés GABAergiques, atténue le syndrome de sevrage alcoolique chez la souris C57BL. Rev Alcool 32: 241-247

Haut Comité de la Santé Publique (1995) La santé en France. La documentation Française, Paris

Le Magnen J, Tran G, Durlach J (1987a) Lack of effects of Ca-acetylhomotaurinate on chronic and acute toxicities of ethanol in rats. Alcohol 4: 103-108

Le Magnen J, Tran G, Durlach J, Martin C (1987b) Dose-dependent suppression of the high alcohol intake of chronically intoxicated rats by Ca-acetylhomotaurinate. Alcohol 4: 97-102

Lhuintre JP, Moore ND, Saligaut C, Boismare F, Daoust M, Chretien P, Tran G, Hillemand B (1985) Ability of calcium bis acetyl homotaurine, a GABA agonist, to prevent relapse in weaned alcoholics. Lancet 4: 1014-1016

Lhuintre JP, Moore ND, Tran G, Steru L, Langrenon S, Daoust M, Parot P, Ladure P, Libert C, Boismare F, Hillemand B (1990) Acamprosate appears to decrease alcohol intake in weaned alcoholics. Alcohol Alcohol 25: 613-622

Paille FM, Guelfi JD, Perkins AC, Royer RJ, Steru L, Parot P (1995) Double-blind randomized multicentre trial of Acamprosate in maintaining abstinence from alcohol. Alcohol Alcohol 30: 239-247

Pelc I, Lebon O, Verbanck P, Lehert P, Opsomer L (1992) Calcium-acetyl-homotaurinate for maintaining abstinence in weaned alcoholic patients: a placebo-controlled double-blind multicenter study. In: Naranjo CA, Sellers E (eds) Novel pharmacologic interventions in alcoholism. Springer, Berlin Heidelberg New York, pp 348-352

World Health Organization (1993) European alcohol action plan. World Health Organization, Copenhagen

Acamprosate Clinical Trials: Methodological Considerations for Assessment of Drinking Behaviour

A.S. Potgieter[1] and P. Lehert[2]

Introduction

Alcohol dependence is a chronic disease in which physical and psychological pathology, addictive behaviour and social influences all interact with treatment to determine the eventual outcome. Despite the complicated nature of these factors, randomised clinical trials remain the standard form of testing a pharmaceutical product for clinical efficacy and safety in this disease, too. However, many mainstays of classical clinical trial design and measurement are lacking or are inappropriate in alcoholism studies. Neither the physical signs of dependence, nor the complications, nor objective markers are ideally suited for regular assessments of change.

The design of randomised trials is primarily influenced by the medical objectives of treatment, including considerations of clinical and statistical appropriateness and regulatory requirements for analysis and presentation of data (Spilker 1991). Clinical trials for psychiatric medication were recently reviewed by Prien and Robinson (1994). Treatment evaluation is progressing from traditional paradigms measuring intake and outcome to expanded paradigms influenced by demographic factors, life context factors, patient treatment experiences and others (Moos et al. 1990). Since no single source of data is free of error, the trend is to use multiple sources of outcome data and seek corroboration (Sobell et al. 1987). Babor et al. (1988) suggested that evaluation of treatment should focus on at least three levels: (1) specific indicators of drinking behaviour, (2) various areas of life functioning and health, and (3) a global dimension of outcome that encompasses drinking behaviour and its consequences and the type of treatment used.

In the clinical trials reviewed in this volume, drinking behaviour was the primary outcome criteria, but treatment effect was also measured by recording associated parameters, including different scales for psychological and physical dependence, severity and nature of dependence (Selzer 1971), social adaptation, rating scales for depression and anxiety (e.g. Hamilton scales; Hamilton 1969), craving assessment by visual analogue scales, laboratory parameters for markers of alcohol consumption or disease and for safety assessment, recording of side effects, concomitant medication, and other routine measures.

[1]Groupe LIPHA, 34, rue St-Romain, 69379 Lyon Cedex 8, France
[2]Department of Statistics, University of Mons, 7000 Mons, Belgium

This chapter attempts to summarise some of the methodological problems related to the measurement and interpretation of drinking behaviour data during long-term treatment for relapse prevention. We make reference to the European-wide clinical research programme with acamprosate, a new drug to maintain abstinence after acute weaning (Zieglgänsberger and Zeise 1992). Different approaches to seek corroboration and better clinical understanding of drinking data are discussed.

Problem Statement

Unstable Symptoms

Most chronic diseases are known for stability in their principal signs or symptoms, and development or progress is measured by incremental changes or lack of change over long periods of time. This stability enhances the validity of individual assessments, and measuring techniques are often adapted to this pattern. However, in alcoholism the principal measure ("symptom") for evaluation of progress (drinking behaviour) could fluctuate between extremes of "complete temporary relief or cure" (abstinence from drinking), to severe worsening (relapse) for any period of time. It is not objective, often not frequent, and with limited validation. Furthermore, unlike subjective assessments of physical symptoms such as pain or psychiatric symptoms such as depression, the alcohol-dependent patient has reasons to minimise or deny the symptoms. The methodologist is hence faced with several crucial problems, including the potential inaccuracy of the measurement, the interpretation of punctual information as a realistic reflection of continuous behaviour for a fluctuating variable, which definitions of therapeutic success to apply and what to consider as the time of "healing", if any. Furthermore, attempts to stabilise the data by experimental design and high frequency of follow-up have not proved beyond doubt that data accuracy for patient declaration is enhanced – while it might improve the "fidelity" of data, it reduces "bandwidth" (Cronbach 1982).

Compliance

Addictive behaviour enhances tendencies to distort the truth about declared behaviour and could negatively affect motivation and compliance; patients might lose interest in being cured and even obstruct progress or assessment. High drop-out rates are common. Missing data, decreasing sample size, in some cases even less than the trial design could foresee and representativity of altered samples often have to be accommodated in the statistical analysis.

Primary Therapy Influence

The primary treatment for alcohol dependence is psycho-social support and counselling, with drug treatment mostly being considered as adjuvant or secondary. Drug trial design should hence consider as primary outcome criteria the measuring of the adjuvant drug effect (mostly blinded), while at the same time assuring (and therefore measuring) equal principal therapy which might or might not have the same duration as the adjuvant therapy. However, due to differences in individual patient psycho-social profiles and variation in psychotherapeutic methodology between therapists, centres, cultures and countries, the standardisation of equal principal therapy to all patients may be a methodological obstacle. The use of treatment manuals is limited in large multicentre trials across cultures, national borders, and different therapeutic approaches.

Sample Size and Trial Duration

High variability and the expected modest success rates, whichever treatment is used, and the phenomenon of limited spontaneous remission requires that trials should be of sufficient size. This could necessitate multicentre trials, but this in itself could increase variability. The addictive and chronic nature of the disease, the natural tendencies for fluctuation of drinking patterns and motivation, and the major influence of social and life events on behaviour and coping mechanisms suggest that long-term trials of at least 6–12 months are advisable if any lasting effects are to be assessed.

Co-morbidity

Co-morbidity and concomitant medication do not only potentially influence treatment and outcome, but could also affect already poorly specific or insensitive laboratory markers such as γ-glutamyl transferase (GGT), aspartate aminotransferase (AST), alanine aminotransferase (ALT) and mean corpuscular volume (MCV). Carbohydrate-deficient transferrin (CDT) might prove to overcome some of the problems of the other markers which suffer from specificity or sensitivity problems.

Frequency of Assessment

Most alcohol treatment centres favour outpatient treatment after and often also during acute detoxification. Patients are seen over long periods of time, in which normal life interacts on the patients and influences outcome. The frequency of follow-up visits could be monthly or even less frequently. Clinical trials which do not reproduce some of these conditions might suffer from restraints on external validity. How to measure drinking behaviour accurately and affordably over extended periods without significant interference with the normal habits and routines of the patients remains a problem. One example is increased patient contact by means of frequent or intruding interviews, contacts or diary cards which could affect outcome by its perceived support to the patient.

Control Groups

Few drugs are available for specific use in alcohol dependence and very few as active control medication in blinded trials. Disulfiram is not ethically accepted by most committees or physicians as blinded medication due to its potentially severe side effects during relapse and if there is no relapse, it is considered by some researchers to be an 'active placebo' (Becker 1979). Different psychotropic medications, including minor tranquilisers, anti-depressants and anti-psychotics have been and are being prescribed in clinical practice as adjuvant therapy, but have not been conclusively shown to attenuate drinking in controlled studies (Miller 1989). Recent research with opioid antagonists showed some efficacy in two short-term trials (O'Malley et al. 1992; Volpicelli et al. 1992); while dopaminergic agents and neuroleptics are under investigation. No medication has as yet been generally accepted or proven to be suited as an active control medication in clinical trials. Placebo control seems the only alternative. However, success attributed to minimal intervention and supportive therapy could potentially enhance the placebo effect.

Drug Safety

Drug safety is routinely assessed by measures including recording of adverse events, laboratory values, and patient assessment during and after withdrawal of study medication. In the treatment of alcohol-dependent patients during and directly after acute detoxification, the effect of the study medication is confounded by prominent and often irregular physical and psychological alcohol withdrawal symptoms and syndromes, craving phenomena, and possible manipulative actions from patients. Low frequency of drug-induced reactions might be masked by this phenomenon. Physical and psychological co-morbidity and complications also contribute to this problem.

Conclusion

The methodology of clinical trials in this field is less standardised than in most other diseases, partly due to the above factors and partly because pharmacotherapy has up to now had limited place in treatment.

Methodological Approaches

External Validity and General Design

Following two pilot studies, the acamprosate clinical research phase was designed to enhance external validity while achieving reasonable sample homogeneity. A large and representative sample was required to be assessed for a long duration to determine both short and long term effects. Eleven double-blind, placebo controlled, multicentre studies were performed in eight European countries on more than 3000 patients. As far as possible, a core protocol was followed in all trials, but with certain variations according to preferences by the participating investigators and also allowing for national and cultural differences. All studies were designed to comply with naturalistic conditions allowing factors outside of treatment to influence the course of treatment, as they would in real life settings (Spilker 1991; Moos et al. 1990). All patients were outpatients, treated according to the routine supportive or psychotherapy offered at the various alcohol treatment centres; they were seen and followed up accordingly, and the blinded study medication was added to the existing treatment in a randomised way.

The period of assessment was between 3 months and 2 years, with an initial double blind medication phase and a subsequent follow-up phase without medication. The shortest trial had a medication phase of 3 months; five trials had medication phases of 6 months and follow-up periods of equal duration (except one with a follow-up phase of 1 month), and five trials had medication phases of 1 year and follow-up periods of equal duration.

All patients were alcohol-dependent according to DSM III or DSM III-R criteria and had at least a 12-month history of alcohol dependence. Patients had to give written informed consent, and had to agree to receive alcohol-weaning therapy during which they had to be abstinent for at least 5 days before the study medication was introduced on the first day after the acute detoxification (weaning) phase.

The following patients were excluded: pregnant women or premenopausal women not practising contraception, and patients with psychiatric disorders which might necessitate specific drug treatment during the weaning or follow-up periods, systemic disease (inadequately controlled diabetes mellitus, hypertension or cardiac failure, septicaemia, active tuberculosis or neoplastic disease), epilepsy unrelated to alcoholism, renal insufficiency or hypercalcaemia of all aetiologies, patients resident in post-cure centres, and patients with no fixed abode.

The following drugs were not allowed: neuroleptics, antidepressants, barbiturates, meprobamate, valproic acid, carbamazepine, clonidine, clomethiazole (apart from weaning period) and all drugs which might influence GGT (with the exception of oral contraceptives). Benzodiazepines were permitted for a period not exceeding 2 weeks following randomisation.

High Drop-out Rate

Sample sizes were in general large enough to accommodate expected high drop out rates. One trial included 62 patients, one 110 patients, and the other nine between 188 and 581 patients (see M. Soyka, this volume).

Patients were to be reached by telephone, or in some trials by letter or home visit in case they dropped out, but, due to the naturalistic model followed in these trials, no extraordinary persuasion or intervention in social activities and conditions beyond what would normally be performed by the treatment centres were required by the protocols.

Reasons for drop-out were recorded as far as possible. Prior to unblinding the treatment code, each patient was assigned a termination status code:

0. Full termination of study period

1.–9. Premature termination of study period for the following reasons:

1. Adverse reactions. Interruption for any adverse event suspected or potentially related to the study medication, treatment or the underlying disease.
2. Concurrent illness. Early termination due to a concurrent illness or adverse event not considered as related to alcoholism or treatment.
3. Death.
4. Serious aggravation of alcoholism which requires withdrawal from protocol (for example for a second inpatient detoxification sequence).
5. Lost to follow-up, without further knowledge of outcome.
6. Protocol violation. Other protocol violations, including breaking the code.
7. Refusal: patient refusal or inability to continue.
8. Overt non-compliance.
9. Concomitant medication. The use of prohibited concomitant medication.

Statistical analyses were performed according to both the intention to treat (ITT) (Gillings and Koch 1991) and the on-treatment (OT) principles. The ITT approach was considered particularly applicable in such trials for alcohol dependence, since the exclusion of drop-outs (predominantly the worst responders) from analysis could introduce a favourable bias to the outcome. Following the ITT principle, any randomised patient who had taken at least one dose of study medication was eligible for analysis (Lehert 1993). Taking the nature of the dependence into consideration, missing data for drinking behaviour (including certain categories of drop-outs) were hence considered as failures of treatment, and where applicable, were equated to non-abstinence. This approach is known to be a strict method of assessing outcome criteria, but is believed to avoid potential bias from OT analysis.

Drinking Behaviour

Relapse was defined as consumption of any alcohol. However, data on severity of relapse, including quantity and frequency of alcohol consumption and duration of drinking periods, were also collected. Relapsing patients could continue the study medication. Drinking behaviour data were based on patient declaration validated by family members or co-habitants where possible.

With reference to the punctual data in this chronic but unstable condition, drinking behaviour analysis attempted to assess the data by different methods exposing different characteristics. The three principal methods were:

1. The relapse rate, categorising patients at each assessment to abstinent, relapse, or absent. This rate was also simplified to a success/failure rate by considering only abstinence as success and presuming absence from assessment, like relapse, as "treatment failure".
2. The time to first relapse.
3. The cumulative abstinence duration (CAD) defined as the total number of days of complete abstinence.

The secondary parameters included:

- Alcohol markers (GGT, MCV, CDT).
- Frequency and quantity of alcohol consumed.
- Physicians clinical global impression and treatment success rate.

Other parameters related to drinking behaviour were:

- Psychological and physiological dependence.
- Psycho-social adaptation.
- Specific physical signs of alcoholism (tremor index/etc.)
- craving for alcohol.

The Relapse Rate at Each Assessment

Transversal assessments (e.g. Chi-square testing) were used, allowing comparison between treatment groups, or even between trials at any assessment interval during treatment (Fig. 1). These were performed on OT and ITT samples. For ITT analysis, the missing values, as for the relapses, were considered in a third category, or equated to treatment failure. Success/failure indexes at different times during treatment can be compiled.

The Time to First Relapse

To introduce the notion of time to the interpretation of the repeated data entries for drinking behaviour during the duration of the trial, the time to first relapse was measured by life-table analysis and survival analysis according to Kaplan-Meier or Lee-Desu (see Fig. 2). The first relapse was considered as a

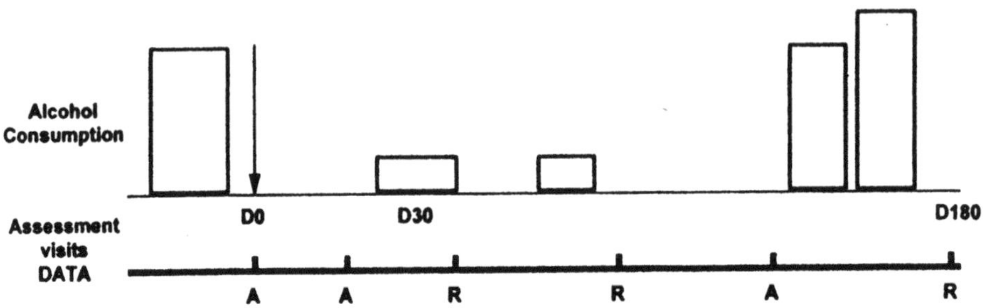

Fig. 1. Relapse rate at each assessment; A = Abstinent, R = Relapse

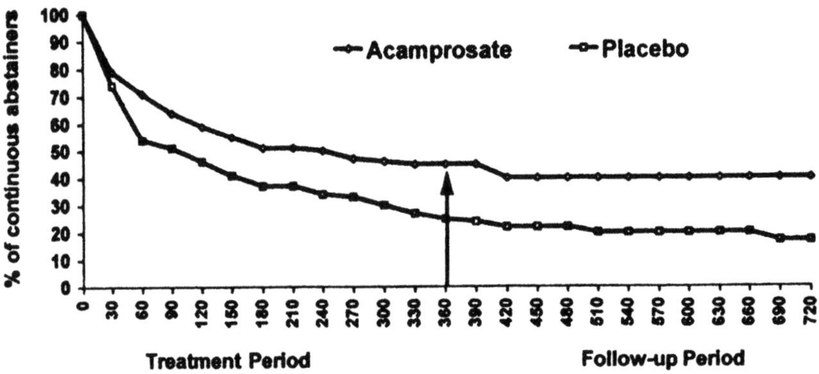

Fig. 2. Assessment of time to first relapse

response. It is possible to censor drop-out patients or to consider them as responders at the time of drop-out. Figure 2 shows the percentage of patients at any time who never had a relapse. Equally, this means that at the end of the graph it could be measured what percentage of patients per treatment group were continuously abstinent throughout the measured period. Another useful comparison is to read off at the middle of the *Y* axis when 50% of patients had their first relapse (i.e. the mean time to first relapse).

The Cumulative Abstinence Duration

We introduced a calculated criterion which could incorporate all relapses and the time factor in one variable: the cumulative abstinence duration (CAD) was defined as the total number of days of abstinence during the period of assessment. It was calculated as the sum of all those periods of complete abstinence, or alternatively as the total period of treatment minus the periods of all relapses (Fig. 3). At each visit the duration of a relapse during the period from the previous to the present visit was recorded. This method is similar to that used in other chronic recidivistic psychiatric conditions where assessment of symptom-free periods are important.

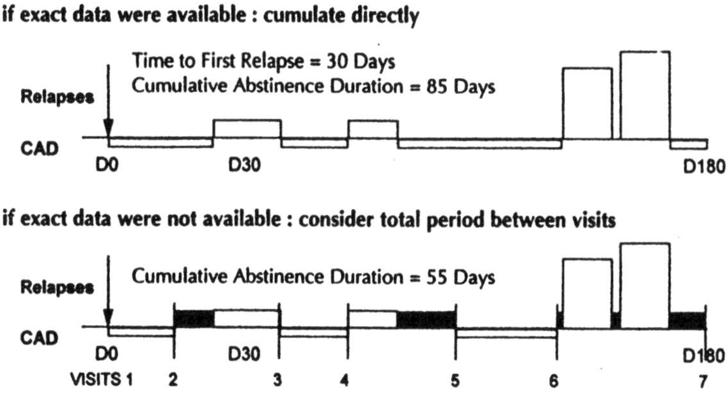

Fig. 3. Cumulative abstinence duration (example of calculation)

One problem encountered in the data was that in certain cases there was incertitude about the exact duration of relapse/s which occurred between two visits. When the relapse period was accurately recorded, it was taken as such. However, where there was uncertainty the most conservative estimate was made: if any relapse was recorded, the total period between the two visits was considered as non-abstinent. In case of patients who dropped out of the study, only the known abstinent days while in the trial were counted. The entire period after drop-out was normally considered as non-abstinent. Due to pronounced top and bottom effects of the data, the Wilcoxon-Mann-Whitney-U test was found more applicable to this data than *t* tests. To assess CAD as a fraction of the potential or real duration of treatment, the corrected cumulative abstinence duration (CCAD) could be calculated, similar to percentage abstinent days. The potential period of treatment was considered as the denominator. That means, the full treatment period for all patients, whether they were retained in the trial or dropped out, except those who withdrew for reasons not related to the underlying illness (concomitant illness unrelated to the treated disease). For example, if a patient was withdrawn for cataract surgery, the potential period of treatment would be considered as only up to the day of withdrawal.

Validation by Laboratory Markers

Standardisation of laboratory values was essential due to the multicentre nature of the trial designs. The method used was to calculate a ratio of the actual laboratory value divided by the laboratory's upper limit of normal (ULN) (Sogliero-Gilbert et al. 1986). The alcohol markers most commonly used were GGT and red cell MCV. Alcohol markers were assessed in all trials and correlated with declared drinking behaviour. Due to known lack of specificity for GGT, investigators took into consideration the absolute GGT value, the previous values of the patient (including baseline), the time between assessment, and other potential causes for elevations. However, this approach was not found practical in assessing large data bases. Hence, before analysing the data, an attempt was made to determine a GGT threshold value that was easily applicable to such data bases and which could indicate a reasonable suspicion of possible relapse (good specificity), without sacrificing too much marker sensitivity, i.e. as conservative as possible. Taking the great variation of GGT and standard laboratory error of 2.0–2.8 SD into account (Whitby et al. 1988), a standardised value of 1.3 times upper limit of laboratory normal was considered by an independent consultant clinical pathologist as a conservative and acceptable level to enhance specificity. Patients equal to or above this level could then be considered as possibly having had a relapse, and below this level were unlikely to have had a relapse. MCV was measured in all patients, and CDT in two trials.

Conclusion

The accurate interpretation of drinking behaviour data over periods of 1 year or more poses particular problems to the clinician and statistician. Data are mostly subjective and not easily verifiable by objective criteria; the measured signs of change are potentially unstable and may fluctuate between extremes of complete abstinence or severe relapse; and the drop-out rate is high resulting in missing data for many patients. A conservative approach to relapse definition and statistical analysis is presented here, and several different methods of interpreting the patterns of drinking were used to obtain a global impression of the drinking behaviour.

To define relapse as any alcohol intake is very conservative. This definition was used mainly since absolute abstinence is still considered the ideal outcome of treatment, and as the data had to be presented to regulatory authorities which prefer conservative assessments. Furthermore, the naturalistic approach to the design of the studies resulted in rather long periods between visits, particularly towards the end of the study periods, which prevented frequent data collection on the exact severity of relapses.

Statistical analysis of only those patients who remain in the trial (OT/per protocol analysis) is expected to introduce a bias in the results. The ITT method was hence considered the most appropriate. The worst case scenario, considering any drop-outs or missing data as non-abstinent, was deemed more appropriate for alcohol dependence than, for example, last observation carried forward (LOCF).

The determination of relapse rates at all visits allowed comparison of drinking behaviour at different periods within one trial or similar periods between different trials. It facilitated pooling of data bases by identifying common time points between different data bases, for example relapse rates in all trials at similar time points, such as at day 30, day 60, etc. The disadvantage of estimating statistical differences at the different intervals is the repetition of the statistical tests which increases the chances of finding a difference (alpha error). Furthermore, testing at each point is independent of the previously measured period, and therefore does not take time or a particular development of a drinking pattern into account.

The survival analysis methodology avoids the above-mentioned alpha error and incorporates time in the assessment. The major disadvantage is that it only considers one aspect of drinking behaviour, in this case the time to first relapse. Once the first relapse occurred, the patient is not considered any more, and it is therefore also a conservative method of analysis, indicating at any time only those patients who had never relapsed. The method is visually presentable and easily interpreted and requires only one statistical test to combine drinking behaviour and time.

The CAD is a measure of the duration of symptom-free periods, whatever the definition of relapse. It appears to be a useful and practical reflection of possible treatment advantage for the patient, the family and the social environment. The CAD is measured in actual days abstinent, rather than a ratio of abstinent over total days treated (percentage of days abstinent), to avoid biased comparison of ratios between different trials of unequal duration. The method of considering all days of a period between two visits as non-abstinent if the actual relapse duration cannot be defined with certainty is conservative, and other possibilities could be investigated. It would, for example, be possible to allocate half of the days between the two visits in such a case, or the known relapse duration plus the days from the reported last day of relapse till the next visit, and similarly for the period after a patient dropped out of the study.

As for all clinical trials, the quality of data is closely related to the trial design. This paper discussed some important restrictions encountered in alcoholism trials and proposed the outline of a multiple method approach to interpreting drinking data. While drinking patterns are day-to-day realisations of patient behaviour, data bases cannot accurately represent this continuum. The presented methodology combined several statistical methods to evaluate different aspects of the same data and thereby construct a multi-facetted clinical reflection of drinking patterns.

References

Babor TF, Dolinsky Z, Rounsaville B, Jaffe J (1988) Unitary versus multidimensional models of alcoholism treatment outcome; an empirical study. J Studies Alcohol 49(2): 167–177

Becker CE (1979) Pharmacotherapy in the treatment of alcoholism. In: Mendelson JH, Mello NK (eds) The diagnosis and treatment of alcoholism. McGraw-Hill, New York

Cronbach LJ (1982) Designing evaluations of educational and social programs. Jossey-Bass, San Francisco

Gillings D, Koch G (1991) The application of the principle of intention to treat to the analysis of clinical trials. Drug Inform J 25: 411-424

Hamilton M (1969) Diagnosis and rating of anxiety. Br J Psychiatr 41: 76–79

Lehert P (1993) Review and discussion of statistical analysis of controlled clinical trials in alcoholism. Alcohol Alcohol 41 [Suppl 2]: 157–163

Miller WR (1989) The addictive behaviours. Treatment of alcoholism, drug abuse, smoking and obesity. Pergamon, Oxford

Moos RH, Finney JW, Cronkite RC (1990) Alcoholism treatment context, process and outcome. Oxford University Press, Oxford

O'Malley SS, Jaffe AJ, Chang G, Schottenfeld RS, Meyer RE, Rounsaville B (1992) Naltrexone and coping skills therapy for alcohol dependence: a controlled study. Arch Gen Psychiatry 49: 881–887
Prien R, Robinson D (eds) (1994) Clinical evaluation of psychotropic drugs: principles and guidelines. Raven, New York
Selzer ML (1971) The Michigan Alcoholism Screening Test: the quest for a new diagnostic instrument. Am J Psychiatr 127: 1653–1658
Sobell MB, Brochu S, Sobell LC, Roy J, Stevens JA (1987) Alcohol treatment outcome evaluation methodology: state of the art 1980–1984. Addict Behav 12: 113–128
Sogliero-Gilbert G, Mosher K, Zubkoff L (1986) Procedures for the simplification and assessment of lab parameters in clinical trials. Drug Inform J 20: 279–296
Spilker B (1991) Guide to clinical trials. Raven, New York
Volpicelli JR, Alterman AI, Hayashida M, O'Brien CP (1992) Naltrexone in the treatment of alcohol dependence. Arch Gen Psychiatry 49: 876–880
Whitby LG, Smith AF, Beckett GJ (1988) Lecture notes on clinical chemistry, 4th edn. Blackwell, Oxford
Zieglgänsberger W, Zeise M (1992) Calcium di-acetylhomotaurinate which prevents relapse in weaned alcoholics decreases the action of excitatory amino acids in neocortical neurons of the rat in vitro. In: Sellers EM, Naranjo CA (eds) Novel pharmacological interventions for alcoholism. Springer, Berlin Heidelberg New York, pp 337–341

Acamprosate in the Treatment of Alcohol Dependence: A 6-Month Postdetoxification Study

I. Pelc[1], O. Le Bon[1], P. Lehert[2], and P. Verbanck[1]

Introduction

Alcohol-dependent patients remain at high risk of relapsing during the first 6 months of the postdetoxification period (Hunt et al. 1971). There is fairly general consensus that the major objectives during this period are the maintenance of abstinence from alcohol (Marlatt and Gordon 1985), the patient's return to a normal life, and preferably his or her establishing stable social and working conditions (Wallace et al. 1988). Many pharmacotherapeutic agents intended to assist the patient through this postdetoxification period are presently under evaluation (Lishow and Goodwin 1987; Litten and Allen 1991; Verbanck et al. 1993). Among them, disulfiram (Fuller et al. 1986), serotonergic agents (Naranjo and Bremner 1992) and naltrexone (Volpicelli et al. 1992; O'Malley et al. 1992) appear to be the most promising. However, the design of the trials performed to test the value of these compounds remained far removed from the "naturalistic" conditions of treatment of most alcoholic patients, and, for this reason, their value in common practice is still unclear.

Acamprosate (Ca-acetyl homotaurinate), a relatively new drug still under evaluation, was reported to reduce alcohol consumption (Le Magnen et al. 1987) and withdrawal symptoms (Gewiss et al. 1991) in drinking animals. There are also some indications that it could reduce alcohol consumption in humans (Lhuintre et al. 1984, 1985, 1990).

The compound is derived from the GABAergic agonist homotaurine (Daoust et al. 1991), and its pharmacological effects, although not yet fully understood, appear to be related to interaction with GABA and excitatory amino-acid systems (Bouchenafa et al. 1990; Zeise et al. 1990).

The objectives of this multicenter study (five centers) were to evaluate some of these ascribed effects of acamprosate over a 6-month postdetoxification period on alcohol-dependent patients, as diagnosed according to the criteria of the third edition of the *Diagnostic and Statistical Manual of Mental Disorders* (*DSM-III*; American Psychiatric Association 1980). The protocol was designed specifically for "natural" conditions (Moos et al. 1990): patients with a prog-

[1]Laboratoire de Psychologie Médicale et Alcoologie, Université Libre de Bruxelles (Campus Brugmann), Place Van Gehuchten, 4, 1020 Brussels, Belgium
[2]Facultés Catholiques de Mons, Département de Sciences Economiques Appliquées, 7000 Mons, Belgium

nosis throughout the complete spectrum from good to bad were included in the cohort, and attendance at follow-up visits relied heavily on the patients' own motivation. Efforts at contacting patients who did not return for follow-up visits were relatively limited. This "natural" approach was preferred for two reasons: (a) to reproduce relatively "realistic" conditions of treatment as we believe are found in the practical situation faced by a large group of physicians in the public and private health domain; this experimental design seemed to us to be most appropriate for determining whether such a drug could be of value in the treatment of alcoholics in common practice; and (b) to investigate whether the drug has an effect on the patient's "spontaneous" tendency to attend the follow-up visits.

The outcome of alcoholic patients lost to follow-up during and after treatment remains uncertain (Alterman et al. 1987). However, we feel that patients lost to follow-up during the early withdrawal phases (up to 6 months after detoxification) should be considered as treatment failure (Edwards 1989; Nathan and Skinstad 1987), and in our data analysis, according to the principles of intention to treat (ITT), these patients were therefore included (Gillings and Koch 1991).

Materials and Methods

Patients and Materials

A total of 104 patients between the ages of 18 and 65 years were included directly or not more than 2 days after a 3-week inpatient acute detoxification period if they conformed to the DSM-III criteria for alcohol dependence, and if their γ-glutamyl transferase (GGT) values were above the upper limits of normal before detoxification. We attempted to evaluate a "natural" group of patients, including those with poor prognosis.

Patient assessment at inclusion and follow-up included:

- Initial diagnostic criteria: DSM-III, CAGE questionnaire (Ewing 1984), previous weaning attempts, demands for help with alcohol-related problems, use of disulfiram or self-help groups, severity of alcohol abuse, awareness of problem and family history
- Biochemical and hematological screening at every visit
- Continual evaluation: alcohol consumption records, psychosocial criteria, psychological and physiological dependence, linear scale for craving, tremors, disorders of sensation (Pelc and Van Wijnsberghe 1988), Hamilton depression and anxiety scales, Clinical Global Impression (CGI), and drug side effects

Study Design and Treatment Regime

A randomized, double-blind (sealed envelopes), parallel, placebo-controlled (identical regimen) study with informed consent and ethical approval was performed. The double-blind status was maintained throughout the treatment period. During the 6-month treatment period the patients received the medication and supportive psychotherapy but no other forms of treatment. In the active group the treatment consisted of two tablets of acamprosate three times a day (each tablet 0.333 g, totalling 1998 g per os per day) in individuals with a body mass of more than 60 kg, and two tablets in the morning, one at lunch time, and one at night in individuals of less than 60 kg body mass (1332 g per day). For the first 2 weeks the patients were seen weekly to establish a routine and thereafter at follow-up visits on days 30, 90, and 180. No disulfiram or psychotropic medication (except chloral hydrate) were permitted.

A CGI evaluation was recorded at each visit. At each visit it was also recorded whether the patient was abstinent or had relapsed. Relapse was defined as the patient's having had any alcohol consumption. In the relapse, patients were advised to continue taking their tablets. If the relapse period exceeded 3–4 days, the patients were to be admitted for classical in-patient detoxification with benzodiazepines for a period not exceeding 14 days and with continuation of administration of the active or placebo tablets. Patients who did not comply with follow-up appointments were contacted by telephone or letter. If these measures failed, the patient was considered as to have dropped out.

Analysis of Data

According to the ITT principle, patients lost to follow-up and those who experienced early termination related to the studied pathology (concomitant medication, refusal to continue, lack of compliance) were included in the analysis as treatment failures. Relapse rate was compared between treatment groups at each examination (Chi square test and survival actuarial technique with relapse as a response, Mantel-Cox test; Cutler and Ederer 1958). To summarize patient performance, the number of abstinence days (cumulative abstinence duration, CAD) was calculated in totalizing the duration of abstinent periods (0 days for non-abstinent periods) and compared by *t* test. Laboratory values (evolution in time) were analyzed according to classical on treatment principles by repeated measurement or analysis of variance.

Results

Of the 104 patients included, two patients were withdrawn during the first 10 days due to unrelated serious illness (malignancy) and the use of disulfiram, respectively. Therefore, 102 patients were eligible for analysis: 47 on placebo and 55 on acamprosate (32 women and 70 men) with a mean age of 42.6 years (s.d. 8.36). At the time of selection and inclusion, the two groups were prac-

Table 1. Baseline comparison data. The AST, ALT, GGT and MCV are expressed in standardized values (i.e. actual value divided by the upper limit of the normal). No significant difference was observed

	Placebo	Acamprosate
Age (years)	43.11 ± 8.90	48.16 ± 7.93
Men (*n*)	33 (70%)	37 (67%)
Women (*n*)	14 (30%)	18 (33%)
AST/ULN (day 0)	1.62 ± 1.84	1.77 ± 2.02
ALT/ULN (day of the selection)	4.83 ± 6.82	5.34 ± 6.84
GGT/ULN (day 0)	2.61 ± 3.99	2.96 ± 3.62
MCV/ULN (day 0)	1.02 ± 0.09	1.02 ± 0.11
Hamilton anxiety score	24.84 ± 3.98	25.18 ± 7.58
Hamilton depression score	16.40 ± 8.39	15.54 ± 1.08

AST, aspartate aminotransferase; ULN, upper limits of normal; ALT, alamine aminotransferase;

tically identical for all variables described, with no statistically significant difference (see Table 1).

Compliance, Abstinence, and Relapse

At each follow-up visit, it was recorded whether a patient was abstinent, had relapsed or was not attending (lost for that examination). Patients lost to follow-up were considered as noncompliant to the treatment program.

At the termination of the follow-up period, 29 out of the 55 patients on active treatment (34%) had dropped out of the treatment program, compared with 37 out of 47 (79%) in the placebo group (p=0.016). (See Fig. 1 and Table 2).

A statistical comparison of relapsers and abstainers suffered from the small numbers after drop out. However, when the dropouts were considered together with the relapsers as treatment failures, a statistically significant difference between active and placebo groups became evident: 64% vs 43% success rate at day 30 (chi square, p=0.031), 42% vs 28% (p=0.132) at day 90, and 33% vs 9% (p=0.003) at day 180.

Applying the survival actuarial technique for evaluation of abstinence (considering relapse or lost to follow-up as reponse) was a rather unforgiving and critical statistical method: only one relapse would irrevocably place the patient in the relapse (failure) category: in the group on active treatment, 13 patients (24%) had remained abstinent throughout the trial, versus 2 (4%) in the placebo group (Mantel Cox, p=0.049).

Another method of assessment used was calculation of the duration of (CAD). Since reported duration of relapse is often unreliable, any relapse between two visits was considered as to have been for the whole period between the two visits (0 days abstinence per relevant period). The CAD was 60.24 days (s.d. 21.55) in the active group and 49.07 (s.d. 14.74) for placebo (t test, p=0.003).

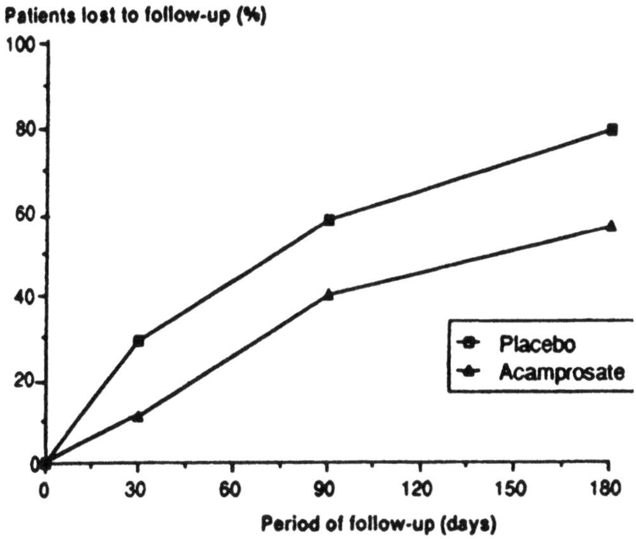

Fig. 1. The proportion of patients who dropped out of the treatment program at each visit during the 6-month observation. The results are expressed in percentage of patients who were included in each treatment group. A significative difference appeared between the placebo and the acamprosate groups since the first visit

γ-Glutamyl Transferase

On treatment statistical analysis of GGT results was performed, but also suffered from the small amount of available data towards the end of trial. In order to be able to compare GGT results from different centers with different reference ranges, the values were mathematically standardized by dividing the actual reported laboratory value by the upper limit of normal (ULN) of the specific laboratory who performed the test; this method was previously described and validated (Sogliero-Gilbert et al. 1986). Therefore a standardized GGT value of 1 would indicate a real GGT value equal to the ULN for that laboratory, a value of 2 signifying double the ULN, etc. Table 3 shows that patients who claimed to be abstinent had returned to and maintained mean GGT values within or close to normal ranges (around 1 or smaller), while the

Table 2. Number of patients who remained abstinent, replapsed, or were lost for follow-up at each visit in both groups. The significance was calculated by the chi-square method

	Day 30		Day 90		Day 180	
	Placebo	Acamprosate	Placebo	Acamprosate	Placebo	Acamprosate
Lost	13 (28%)	7 (13%)	26 (55%)	21 (38%)	37 (79%)	31 (56%)
Relapse	14 (30%)	13 (24%)	8 (17%)	11 (20%)	6 (13%)	6 (11%)
Abstain	20 (42%)	35 (63%)	13 (28%)	23 (42%)	4 (9%)	18 (33%)
n	47	55	47	55	47	55
	$p<0.068$		$p<0.202$		$p<0.012$	

Table 3. Evolution of the γ-glutamyl transferease (GGT) values for the patients who were considered to relapse or to remain abstinent at each visit. The GGT are expressed in standardised values. The sigificance was calculated by the t test

	Day 30		Day 90		Day 180	
	Mean ± SD	*n*	Mean ± SD	*n*	Mean ± SD	*n*
Relapse	2.10 ± 1.83	22	1.72 ± 1.41	8	2.42 ± 2.01	4
Abstain	0.75 ± 0.69	51	0.79 ± 0.78	34	1.40 ± 2.07	17
$p <$	0.001		0.001		0.001	

relapsers had mean values 2–3 times higher than the laboratory ULN, supporting patient claims of abstinence.

When possible, the ratio between a patient's GGT at a specific visit and his/her own value at day 0 was also calculated (GGT at visit x /GGT at day 0; Table 4).

Clinical Global Impression

A CGI scale was recorded at each visit. This standardized rating scale is a five-level instrument (the levels being: much worse, worse, stable, better, or much better) comparing the patient's overall clinical status at each evaluation with his/her status at intake (Guy 1976; Guy and Bonato 1970). In line with the ITT principle of including all patients, those in the first three categories and all patients lost to follow-up were considered as treatment failures. Patients in the last two categories were considered as treatment successes. At the end of trial, 17 patients on active treatment (31%) and six on placebo (13%) had improved (chi-square, p=0.027; see Table 5).

Other Criteria Applied

No significant statistical differences between the two groups could be detected for the other criteria evaluated, for example, Hamilton anxiety (p=0.581), psychological dependence (p=0.299), physiological dependence (p=0.275), other laboratory investigations, or any physical parameters (p values refer to calculations for day 180).

Table 4. Evolution of the γ-glutamyl transferease (GGT) ratio (GGT at visit × / GGT at day 0) in both groups of patients at each visit. The significance was calculated by the t test

	Day 30		Day 90		Day 180	
	Mean ± SD	*n*	Mean ± SD	*n*	Mean ± SD	*n*
Placebo	1.55 ± 1.71	30	1.35 ± 1.30	16	2.52 ± 2.44	6
Acamprosate	0.88 ± 1.12	43	0.70 ± 0.55	25	1.22 ± 1.83	15
$p <$	0.01		0.01		0.01	

Table 5. Evolution of the clinical global impression at each visit. The significance was calculated by the chi-square method

	Day 30		Day 90		Day 180	
	Placebo	Acamprosate	Placebo	Acamprosate	Placebo	Acamprosate
Failure	21 (45%)	13 (24%)	30 (64%)	26 (47%)	41 (87%)	38 (68%)
Success	26 (55%)	42 (76%)	17 (36%)	29 (53%)	6 (13%)	17 (31%)
$p <$	0.023		0.090		0.027	

Side Effects

Spontaneous complaints were recorded at each visit, and thereafter the investigators made specific enquiries completing a 45-item checklist of possible other symptoms. These did however include many known chronic withdrawal phenomena, and a clear distinction from adverse events was sometimes difficult. Since most adverse events were reported before day 30, and to preserve a maximum number of patients in the analysis, we have summarized those adverse events which occurred in more than 5% in at least one treatment group during the first 30 days (see Table 6). During the early phase of treatment, there was a trend to more gastrointestinal symptoms and headache in the active group, but the statistical threshold was not reached.

To evaluate the complete period of treatment, survival analysis was applied to each adverse event individually from day 0 until day 180, by considering adverse event occurrence as a response. This method was also unable to detect any statistically significant difference between treatment groups.

Discussion

The results of this study reflect the outcome of a natural research methodology on a rather nonintrusive, pragmatic follow-up program. We did not exclude poor prognosis cases such as patients with long histories of alcohol dependence or multiple previous relapses since we believe that our inclusion criteria reflect more truly the patient profile actually encountered by the majority of alcoholic treatment units and private practitioners. We also minimized interference with the patients' lives and normal tendencies to comply or not comply with follow-

Table 6. Adverse events reported at day 30. Only the adverse events reported with more than 5% occurrence in at least one group were presented

Adverse event	Placebo (n=34)	Acamprosate (n=48)
Headaches	4 (12%)	11 (23%)
Memory disturbance	8 (24%)	12 (25%)
Gastralgia	3 (9%)	7 (15%)
Diarrhoea	1 (3%)	5 (15%)
Sweating	6 (18%)	13 (27%)
Sleep disturbance	6 (18%)	12 (25%)

up instructions for two additional and pertinent reasons: to avoid possible bias due to enhanced patient contact (Sobell and Sobell 1980), to evaluate whether or not this drug might have an influence on the patients' compliance to remain in the postdetoxification treatment regime (a form of "drug-related compliance"?).

Poor compliance in alcoholic treatment programs presents a considerable problem for data analysis, as is well-known to most investigators in this field (Nordström and Berglund 1986). Failure to account for dropouts in the "efficacy analyzable population" type of analysis may and often does introduce unfair positive bias to outcome estimates (Edwards 1989; Nathan and Skinstad 1987), and the application of ITT principles has gained increasing acceptance by clinicians (Gillings and Koch 1991). In the light of the specific circumstances of relatively predictable outcome in patients lost during the early stages of treatment of alcohol dependence, and according to the general hypothesis of our study, we decided to apply this method of analysis and therefore considered cases lost to follow-up as treatment failures.

Successful treatment was primarily defined as a patient who completed follow-up and remained abstinent. Over the 6-month follow-up period, it was found that 13 out of 55 patients on active treatment remained completely abstinent throughout treatment, compared with two out of 46 in the placebo group. This appears to be in keeping with previously published studies investigating this drug (Lhuintre et al. 1984, 1985, 1990). The mean cumulative duration of abstinence was longer in the active than in the placebo group (60.24 vs 49.07 days) and relapse occurred considerably later in the active group. GGT values appeared to support the self reports of the patients. The active group also had a higher success rate in the evaluation of overall clinical impression (CGI scale), as assessed by the treating (but "blinded") physicians.

Another interesting result was a considerably better adherence to treatment schedule by the active group, where 44% remained in treatment compared with 21% in the placebo group. In seeking increased aftercare compliance, it appears that voluntary patient cooperation rather than techniques of imposed avoidance are favored by many therapists (Gilbert 1987). This approach probably conforms with the Alcoholics Anonymous viewpoint that, for increased compliance to lead to better outcome, "attraction" efforts to make the patient "keep coming back" are more favored than "promotion" methods. In our study, patients had a relatively free choice to "come back" or not. We hypothesize that the better compliance we found in the active group could be due to a combination of factors amongst which are: a possible reduction in craving, reduction in "loss of control" and interest in alcohol (Lhuintre et al. 1985), as well as less severe withdrawal symptoms (Gewiss et al. 1991) and confirmed better performance on the CGI scale. We further hypothesize that a combination of all these factors perhaps contributed to a better state of general well being (Pelc and Van Wijnsberghe 1988) in the patients on active treatment, and that this improved general well being might have contributed to the better compliance. In our opinion, this apparent tendency in alcohol-dependent patients to actually comply with attempted treatment is promising and deserves further investigation.

It remains difficult to predict outcome of those alcoholics who are lost to follow-up after treatment, particularly long-term (Cross et al. 1990; Mackenzie et al. 1987). Vaillant has emphasized the temporal perspective and the effects that life structure might have upon the cycles of abstention and relapse over many years (Vaillant 1988). However, projections of outcome when patients abscond from the early phases of treatment (weaning and early post detoxification phases) seems less controversial. These losses are more likely to have a negative treatment outcome (Nathan and Skinstad 1987; Hill and Blane 1967; Moss and Bliss 1978; Elal-Lawrence et al. 1987) and are frequently regarded as treatment failures (Edwards 1989; Nathan and Skinstad 1987), with many factors contributing to relapse during this early period (Marlatt and Gordon 1985; Edwards 1989; Vaillant 1988; Elal-Lawrence et al. 1987; De Soto et al. 1989). In our study, we accordingly considered drop-outs as such.

We conclude that acamprosate appeared to have had a statistically significant beneficial effect on important parameters evaluated in this study under naturalistic conditions: total alcohol abstinence, mean period of abstinence, clinical global outcome and degree of compliance. All these are relevant criteria of outcome evaluation in patients with a high risk of relapse.

Further studies on larger groups of patients are needed to confirm that acamprosate makes this probable pharmacotherapeutic contribution in maintaining abstinence after acute withdrawal treatment, and also to identify its specific mechanisms of action on the pathophysiology of alcohol dependence.

References

Alterman AI, Hayashida M, O'Brien CP (1987) Treatment response and safety of ambulatory medical detoxication. J Stud Alcohol 49(2): 160–166

American Psychiatric Association (1980) Diagnostic and statistical manual for mental disorders, 3rd edn. APA, Washington DC

Bouchenafa O, Cwynarski K, Littleton JM (1990) Interactions between excitatory aminoacids and AOTAL in a cell culture model of ethanol dependence. 5th Congress of the International Society of Biomedical Research on Alcoholism 1990; abstract book, abstract 30

Cross GM, Morgan CW, Mooney AJ, Martin CA, Rafter JA (1990) Alcoholism treatment: a ten year study. Alcohol Clin Exp Res 14(2): 169–173

Cutler SJ, Ederer F (1958) Maximum utilization of the life-talk method in analyzing survival. Chron Dis 8: 699–713

Daoust M, Chabenat C, Boucly P (1991) Acamprosate calcium. Drugs Today 27(3): 75–76

De Soto CB, O'Donnel WE, De Soto JL (1989) Long term recovery in alcoholics, Alcohol Clin Exp Res 13(5): 693–697

Edwards G (1989) As the years go rolling by. Drinking problems in time dimension. Bri J Psychiatry 154: 18–26

Elal-Lawrence G, Slade P, Dewey ME (1987) Treatment and follow-up variables discriminating abstainers, controlled drinkers and relapsers. J Stud Alcohol 48(1): 39–49

Ewing JA (1984) Detecting alcoholism: the CAGE questionnaire. J Am Med Assoc 252: 1905–1907

Gewiss M, Heidbredder C, Opsomer L, Durbin P, De Witte P (1991) Acamprosate and diazepam differentially modulate alcohol-induced behavioural and cortical alterations in rats following chronic inhalation of ethanol vapour. Alcohol Alcohol 26 (2): 129–137

Gilbert FS (1987) The effect of aftercare follow-up on treatment outcome among alcoholics. J Stud Alcohol 49(2): 149–159

Gillings D, Koch G (1991) The application of intention-to-treat to the analysis of clinical trials. Drug Inform J 25: 411–424

Guy W(ed) (1976) ECDEU assessment manual for psychopharmacology, 3rd edn. National Institute of Mental Health, Bethesda, MD
Guy W, Bonato RB (eds) (1970) Manual for the ECDEU assessment battery, 2nd edn. National Institute of Mental health, Bethesda, MD
Hill MJ, Blane HT (1967) Evaluation of psychotherapy with alcoholics: a critical review. Q J Stud Alcohol 28: 76–104
Hillemand B, Joly JP, Lhuintre JP, Libert C (1986) Prospects of the management of alcoholism. Part 1: generalities and models of therapeutic relations with the alcoholic patient. Part 2: the alcohol-dependent person's itinerary towards regained freedom. Sem Hop Paris 62: 3391-3395, 3468-3474
Hillemand B, Lhuintre JP, Steru L, Daoust M, Moore N (1989) Essai thérapeutique multicentrique du N bis acétylhomotaurinate de calcium (Ca Aota) dans le traitment de l'alcoolo-dépendant. Rev Alcool 34(1): 9–28
Hunt WA, Barnett W, Branch LG (1971) Relapse rates in addiction programs. J Clin Psychol 27: 455–456
Le Magnen J, Tran G, Durlach J, Martin C (1987) Dose dependent suppresion of the high alcohol intake of chronically intoxicated rats by Ca-acetylhomotaurinate. Alcohol 4: 97–102
Lhuintre JP, Daoust M, Tran G, Moore N, Chretien P, Hillemand B, Boismare F (1984) Calcium acetyl-homotaurinate (Ca-aota) reduces alcohol consumption by ethilics. Alcohol Clin 8: 103
Lhuintre JP, Daoust M, Moore N, Chretien P, Saligaut C, Tran G, Boismare F, Hillemand B (1985) Ability of calcium bis homotaurinate, a GABA-agonist, to prevent relapse in weaned alcoholics. Lancet I: 1014–1016
Lhuintre JP, Moore N, Tran G, Steru L, Langrenon S, Daoust M, Parot P, Ladure P, Libert C, Boismare F, Hillemand B (1990) Acamprosate appears to decrease alcohol intake in weaned alcoholics. Alcohol (1987) Alcohol 25(6): 613–622
Liskow BI, Goodwin DW (1987) Pharmacological treatment of alcohol intoxication, withdrawal and dependence: a critical review. J Stud Alcohol 48(4): 356–370
Litten RZ, Allen JP (1991) Pharmacotherapies for alcoholism: promising agents and clinical issues. Alcohol Clin Exp Res 15 (4): 620–633
MacKenzie A, Funderburk FR, Allen RP, Stefan RL (1987) The characteristics of alcoholics frequently lost to follow-up. J Stud Alcohol 48(2): 119–123
Marlatt GA, Gordon JR (1985) Relapse prevention: maintenance strategies in the treatment of addictive behaviours. Guilford, New York
Moos RH, Bliss F (1978) Difficulty of follow-up and outcome of alcoholism treatment. J Stud Alcohol 39: 473–481
Moos RH, Finney JW, Cronkite RC (1990) Alcoholism treatment: context, process, and outcome. Oxford University Press, Oxford
Naranjo CA, Sellers EM, Lawrin MO (1986) Modulation of ethanol intake by serotonin uptake inhibitors. J Clin Psychiatry 47 [Suppl]: 16–20
Naranjo CA, Sellers EM, Sullivan JT, Woodley DV, Kadlec K, Sykora K (1987) The serotonin uptake inhibitor citalopram attenuates ethanol intake. Clin Pharmacol Ther 41: 266–274.
Nathan PE, Skinstad A-H (1987) Outcomes of treatment for alcohol problems: cuirrent methods, problems and results. J Consult Clin Psychol 55(3): 332–340
Nordström G, Berglund M (1986) Successfully adjusted alcoholics lost to long-term follow-up. A prospective study. Drug Alcohol Depend 18: 116–122
Pelc I, Van Wijnsberghe J (1988) Nouveaux éléments pour une thérapie dynamico-comportementale de l'alcoolisme. Actual Psychiatri 7: 78–82
Sobell LC, Sobell MB (1980) Frequent follow-up as data gathering and continued care with alcoholics. Int J Addict 16: 1077–1086
Sogliero-Gilbert G, Mosher K, Zubkoff A (1986) Procedure for the simplification and assessment of lab parameters in clinical trials. Drug Inform J 20: 279–296
Vaillant GE (1988) What can long-term follow-up teach us about relapse and prevention of relapse in addiction. Br J Addict 83: 1147–1157
Verbanck P, Barrias J, Besson J, Borg S (1993) Pharmacological approach of the treatment of drinking problems: a critical overview. Alcohol Alcohol [Suppl 2]: 139–144
Waisberg JL (1990) Patient characteristics and outcome of inpatient treatment for alcoholism. Adv Alcohol Subst Abuse 8(3/4): 9–32
Wallace J, McNeil D, Gilfillan D, MacLean K, Fanella F (1988) Six month treatment outcomes in socially stable alcoholics: abstinence rates. J Subst Abuse Treat 5: 247–252
Zeise ML, Kasparow S, Capogna M, Zieglgänsberger W (1990) Calciumdiacetylhomotaurinate (Ca-aota) decreases the action of excitatory amino acids in the rat neocortex in vitro. Prog Clin Biol Res 351: 237–242

Contribution of Acamprosate in Maintaining Abstinence in Weaned Alcohol-Dependent Patients: Additional Results of the Second French Multicentre Study

F. Paille[1], P. Parot[2], and C. Gillet[1]

Acamprosate is a synthetic compound derived from homotaurine and has been marketed in France since 1989 to maintain abstinence in weaned alcohol-dependent subjects. Its efficacy for this indication has been demonstrated in previous studies (Lhuintre et al. 1985, 1990; Pelc et al. 1992), and the results of our study were published in 1995 (Paille et al. 1995). A more detailed analysis of our data with a number of additional findings concerning duration of abstinence, evolution of drinking behaviour, and prognostic criteria for better outcomes are reported and discussed in this article.

Patients and Methods

Patient Selection and Eligibility

Alcohol-dependent patients, defined according to the DSM-III-R criteria, between 18 and 65 years, were enrolled by 31 specialised alcohol treatment centres. They had to give written informed consent to participate in this 18-month study as outpatients, to undergo detoxification treatment, and be motivated to remain abstinent. Additional selection criteria included either a gamma-glutamyl transferase (GGT) level at least twice the upper limit of the normal ranges and/or a mean red cell corpuscular volume (MCV) greater than 98 fl, which provided evidence of current alcohol consumption during the pre-inclusion assessment period. Patients without a fixed address, patients with a severe psychiatric or organic disease, pregnant or breast-feeding women, patients taking a nonpermitted concomitant medication or who had three weaning attempts in the previous 2 years were excluded.

[1]Centre d'Alcoologie, Hôpital Fournier, 36 quai de la Bataille, 54035 Nancy Cedex, France
[2]Pharmaceutical Consultant, 12, avenue G.Pompidou, 92800 Puteaux, France

Treatment Phase

The study treatment started after a detoxification period of 7–28 days. Eligible patients were randomly assigned to three different groups:

- Group I, placebo group (n=179), six tablets of placebo daily;
- Group II, acamprosate 1.3 g/day group (n=188), four tablets of acamprosate and two tablets of placebo daily;
- Group III, acamprosate 2 g/day group (n=173), six tablets of acamprosate daily.

The study medication was given double-blind for 12 months, after which acamprosate was withdrawn and replaced in all three groups by placebo for an additional 6-month period, without the patients' knowledge of this.

On Day 0 (beginning of the treatment period), drinking history was recorded, states of anxiety and depression were scored using the Covi (Covi and Lipman 1984) and Raskin (Raskin et al. 1969) scales, as well as quality of life (according to the Spitzer QL index), craving for alcohol (rated as none, controlled, uncontrolled), and dependence as clinically assessed by the investigator (according to the Le Gô scale).

Patients were evaluated every month for the first 6 months, and every 2 months for a further 12 months. At each evaluation, the investigator recorded the number of drinking days reported by the patient since the last visit, the quantity and the frequency of his alcohol consumption, his craving for alcohol and his level of anxiety and depression. Laboratory criteria for efficacy and safety including GGT, alanine and aspartate aminotransferases (ASAT and ALAT), blood alcohol level, and MCV were collected at 3, 6, 12, and 18 months by a single laboratory. Quality of life was evaluated at 6 and 12 months. The safety of the product was assessed at each visit by the clinician, and patients were asked to complete a monthly self-evaluation questionnaire.

All patients received unstructured supportive psychotherapy throughout the study. Concomitant medication was monitored and recorded. Psychotropic treatments were only prescribed exceptionally and for short periods: maprotiline was allowed as antidepressant and lorazepam as anxiolytic. Somatic treatments initiated more than 3 months prior to the study were permitted.

Treatment compliance was assessed from tablet counts at each visit. When a patient failed to take the study treatment for more than 30 days, he/she was withdrawn from the trial.

Outcome Measures

The main efficacy criterion adopted was continuous abstinence rate at 6 and 12 months. Secondary criteria included time to first relapse, cumulated abstinence duration, alcohol craving, product safety assessed on the basis of clinical and laboratory data, clinician's global impression, and treatment compliance. To better characterise the abstinence, a more in-depth analysis was performed to assess the longest period of abstinence, the evolution of drinking behaviour, and the prognostic criteria for better outcomes.

Statistical Analysis

The high drop-out rate from long-term studies in the field of alcoholism and the potential risk of patients remaining in the study being at variance from the baseline population ruled out a simple data analysis on patients who completed the study (Lehert 1993). An intention-to-treat analysis was therefore performed: all randomised patients who had taken the treatment at least once were analysed in terms of success or failure. Patients who prematurely withdrew from the study were considered as treatment failures. Only patients who consumed no alcohol at all were classified as a successful outcome of treatment.

The statistical analysis was carried out using SPSS software, version 4. The simplest statistical tests were used for enumerations and means for the description of the discontinuous and continuous variables. The chi-square test and one-way analysis of variance, or the Mann-Whitney U test were used for the comparison of the same variables.

Results

Sample Description

A total of 538 patients, with a mean age of 43.2±8.6 years, were randomised to the three treatment groups. Most of them (80%) had undergone detoxification in hospital, and one patient out of two was being treated for the first time. A description of the whole population is given in Tables 1 and 2. No statistically significant differences were found between the three groups on any of the variables. Since patients with severe psychiatric disorders had been excluded, there was no marked anxiety or depression as shown by the mean scores on the Covi and Raskin scales (anxiety, 5.6±2.7; depression, 4.4±2.9; scales calibrated from 0 to 12).

Clinic Attendance

At the end of the first year of treatment, 55.9% of the patients had dropped out of the study and 13.9% of them were lost to follow up. Acamprosate appeared to induce a dose-dependent improvement in the duration of patient follow-up. At 12 months, in fact, 35.0% of patients remained in the placebo group, as opposed to 45.2% in the group on 1.3 g/day of acamprosate, and 52% in the group on 2 g/day ($p=0.005$; Table 3). Similarly, patients of 2 g/day of acamprosate were followed-up for an additional 75 days compared with patients on placebo ($p=0.006$).

A profile study of patients showed that those who were lost to follow-up or who refused to continue the study treatment tended to be younger than patients who completed the study (25.2% vs. 10.6% aged between 25 and 34 years); they less often lived with their families (64.1% vs. 82.3%) and were more often employed (74.6% vs. 67.2%; Table 4). Their drinking history was similar,

Table 1. Description of the population: sociodemographic characteristics, anxiety, depression and quality of life

Variable	Placebo (n=177)	Acamprosate 1.3g/day (n=188)	Acamprosate 2g/day (n=173)	Total	Significance (p)
Age (years)	42.5±8.9	43.7±8.6	43.3±8.3	43.2±8.6	0.428
Sex					
Males	147	146	137	430	
Females	30	42	36	108	0.420
Height(cm)	171.5±7.7	170.2±8.0	169.5±9.2	170.4±8.3	0.084
Weight (kg)	70.9±12.9	69.3±13.9	67.7±11.5	69.3±12.9	0.078
Living conditions					
Alone	37	38	35	110	
With family	131	145	133	409	0.630
In home/hotel	9	5	4	18	
Employment status					
Employed	115	138	114	367	0.617
Other	62	50	58	170	
Covi anxiety scale score before detoxification	5.9±2.6	5.4±2.6	5.5±2.8	5.6±2.7	0.192
Raskin depression scale score before detoxification	4.6±2.85	4.4±2.9	4.2±2.9	4.4±2.9	0.494
Quality of life	6.45±2.0	6.5±9.0	6.3±2.3	6.4±2.1	0.734

except for the duration of abstinence after the last detoxification period which was shorter in the group lost to follow-up (54.9% vs. 44.9% presented a period of abstinence shorter than 5 months after the last detoxification). At baseline, the scores of anxiety and depression and the level of alcohol dependence were lower in patients lost to follow-up than in patients who completed the study: 30.1% of the patients lost to follow-up had a Covi score ≤3 vs. 24.7% of those

Table 2. Description of the population: drinking behaviour

Variable	Placebo (n=177)	Acamprosate 1.3g/day (n=188)	Acamprosate 2g/day (n=173)	Total	Significance (p)
Alcohol comsumption (g/day)	192±108	189±161	180±89.5	187±124	0.652
Duration (years)	8.5±6.5	9.8±7.7	10.1±7.1	9.5±7.1	0.093
Craving					
None	0	1	0	1	
Controlled	51	65	54	170	0.512
Uncontrolled	98	95	95	288	
Method of detoxification					
Outpatient	41	41	35	117	0.801
Inpatient	136	147	138	421	

Table 3. Percentage of patients remaining in the trial at different assessments

Assessment	Placebo (n=177) %	Acamprosate 1.3 g/day (n=188) %	Acamprosate 2 g/day (n=173) %	Significance (p)
Day 90	75.7	77.7	81.5	0.41
Day 180	52.5	58.5	70.5	0.002
Day 360	35.0	45.2	52.0	0.005
Day 540	29.9	37.2	43.4	0.034

Table 4. Baseline predictive factors for early treatment termination

Variable	Normal termination (%)	Relapse (%)	Lost to follow-up or refused to continue (%)	Other reasons (%)
Age				
25–34	10.6	11.2	25.2	12.3
35–44	42.9	44	55.2	44.4
45–54	30.3	31	16.8	21
>54	16.2	13.8	2.8	22.2
Living conditions				
With family	82.3	77.6	64.1	80.2
Other	17.7	22.4	35.9	19.8
Employment status				
In work	67.2	68.1	74.6	60.5
Other	32.8	31.9	25.4	39.5
Alcohol consumption (g/day)				
0–99	13.7	7.8	9.1	8.6
100–200	59.4	56.5	63.6	66.7
>200	26.9	35.7	27.3	24.7
Period of abstinence after last detoxification				
0–5 months	44.9	41.9	54.9	44.1
6–11 months	27.6	25.8	18.3	26.5
>12 months	27.6	32.3	26.8	29.4
Covi score				
0–3	24.7	19	30.1	17.5
4–6	34.3	38.8	35	38.8
7–9	38.4	35.3	30.8	35
10–12	2.5	6.9	4.2	8.7
Raskin score				
0–4	53.5	49.1	49	43.2
5–8	38.4	40.5	43.4	46.9
9–12	8.1	10.3	7.7	9.9
Quality of life score				
0–3	10.2	9.6	5.6	9.9
4–7	56.9	60.9	60.8	58
8–10	33	29.6	33.6	32.1

who completed the study. The quality of life was better in early terminators (only 5.6% of them had a score ≤3 vs. 10.2% of those who completed the study).

Abstinence

Number of Patients Continuously Abstinent

At each visit, the percentage of patients maintaining continuous abstinence from the beginning of the study treatment was higher in the group on 2 g/day of acamprosate than in the placebo group. The difference was statistically significant at 6 months (p=0.018), but not at 12 months (p=0.096) (Table 5). The results obtained with the low dose of acamprosate (1.3 g/day) came in between.

Duration of Abstinence

The number of days of abstinence during the length of the study was assessed according to the following three criteria.

Duration of Continuous Abstinence. The mean number of days of continuous abstinence (or time to the first relapse after detoxification) was significantly longer in the group on 2 g/day of acamprosate than in the placebo group (153 days±197 vs. 102 days±165; p=0.005). The group on 1.3 g/day of acamprosate was between the two (135 days±189). Intergroup differences were not significant, but the global analysis nevertheless confirmed that acamprosate prolonged the initial period of abstinence (p=0.032).

Longest Period of Abstinence. A total of 24% of the whole population relapsed before day 30. Relapse occurred more frequently in the placebo group (31.1%) than in the group on 2 g/day of acamprosate (16.8%). The mean longest period of abstinence was significantly shorter in the placebo group (130 days±172) than in the group on 1.3 g/day of acamprosate (172 days±190; p=0.020) and in the group on 2 g/day of acamprosate (191 days±196; p=0.001). On the other hand, there was no statistical difference between the two acamprosate groups. For the whole population, in 48.9% of the cases the longest period of abstinence

Table 5. Percentage of patients who maintained continuous abstinence

Assessment	Placebo (n=177) %	Acamprosate 1.3g/day (n=188) %	Acamprosate 2g/day (n=173) %	Significance (p)
Day 90	33.3	39.4	41	0.29
Day 180	18.6	26.6	31.8	0.018
Day 360	11.3	18.1	19.1	0.096
Day 540	9	10.6	14.5	0.26

started on day 0, with a higher frequency in the group on 2 g/day of acamprosate (57.2%) than in the placebo group (42.4%).

Cumulative Period of Abstinence. The cumulative period of abstinence is defined as the total number of days of abstinence, whether continuous or not, during the 1-year treatment period. Patients who did not attend a visit were assumed to have been drinking since the last assessment. The mean cumulative duration of abstinence was 173 days±126 for the placebo group, 198 days±133 for the group on 1.3 g/day of acamprosate, and 223 days±134 for the group on 2 g/day of acamprosate. The difference between the placebo group and the group on 2 g/day of acamprosate was highly significant (p=0.0005), while the difference between the placebo group and the group on 1.3 g/day of acamprosate was near statistical significance (p=0.055).

Evolution of Drinking Behaviours During the Course of the Study

The assessment of drinking behaviour from one visit to the next confirmed the patients in the acamprosate groups remained more abstinent than in the placebo group, with a proportion of abstinent patients significantly higher at every evaluation, except at 3 months. At 6 months, 44.5% of the patients in the group on 2 g/day of acamprosate, 38.8% in the group on 1.3 g/day of acamprosate, and 29.9% in the placebo group were abstinent (p<0.001). At 12 months, the proportions were 34.7%, 27.7%, and 18.6% respectively (p<0.001).

The analysis of patients who were abstinent at 12 months but had consumed alcohol at the time of interim visits showed a shorter duration of alcohol consumption in patients on 2 g/day of acamprosate: 33% of them had been drinking for less than 1 month during the 1-year treatment, as opposed to 24% of those on placebo.

Moreover, when looking at patients whose consumption was rated as controlled (≤40 g/day of pure alcohol), patients on 2 g/day of acamprosate tended to control their consumption more frequently than those on placebo or, even better, when back to abstinence (78.7% compared with 68.9%). However, the difference was not statistically significant. On the other hand, 74.3% of the patients treated with the high dose of acamprosate and whose alcohol consumption was not controlled at one visit had returned to controlled consumption or abstinence at the next visit, as opposed to 59.1% only in the placebo group (p=0.04).

Craving for Alcohol

At baseline, all patients but one presented a craving for alcohol that 62.7% of them declared uncontrollable. Despite a steadily higher proportion of patients with no – or only a weak – craving for alcohol in the group on 2 g/day of acamprosate, there was no significant difference between the groups, except at 3 months (placebo group, 39.6%; acamprosate 2 g/day group, 59.4%; p=0.015).

Baseline craving was not a predictor of early study termination as it was identical between patients who completed the trial normally and those who prematurely left the trial (relapsers or lost to follow-up patients).

Clinical Findings

From a clinical point of view, the main findings were a gradual improvement of the general condition (mean weight gain of 2–2.5 kg) in all three groups. Among physical signs of alcohol consumption according to the Le Gô scale, only tremor was significantly less marked in the acamprosate 2 g/day group than in the placebo group, between the 3rd and 12th month. The scores on the Covi and Raskin scales fell gradually during the course of the study, but there was no statistically significant difference between groups.

As for the global clinical impression expressed by the investigators, the disease at the start of detoxification was assessed as moderate to very severe in nearly all patients (97.8%). At 3 months, all groups had improved. The high-dose acamprosate group, however, had improved more significantly than the placebo group: 40.9% of patients on placebo were still classified as moderately to extremely ill against 31.4% only in the group on 2 g/day of acamprosate (p=0.029). At 12 months, the percentage of these patients was 31.7% in the placebo group and 13.7% in the high-dose acamprosate group (p=0.041).

Laboratory Assessments

The evolution in the biological markers was not very meaningful, although it should be emphasised that laboratory variables could only be measured for patients remaining in the study. In terms of mean values, no significant difference was observed for any marker of drinking, even after log transformation. However, the percentage of patients presenting a GGT level within laboratory's normal range was significantly higher in the acamprosate groups than in the placebo group, at six months (42.8% vs. 29.4%; p=0.011) and at 12 months (35.3% vs. 21.5%; p=0.015). This was also true for blood alcohol level and ASAT.

Prognostic Criteria for Better Outcomes, Regardless of the Study Treatment

Possible links between initial sociodemographic data, alcohol history, study treatment and outcome criteria were studied. Results were classified as follows: patients were considered a success when abstinent at 6 and 12 months (responders, 24.2%); a partial success when abstinent at one of the two visits only (partial responders, 16.4%), and a failure when not abstinent at either of these visits (nonresponders, 59.5%).

The failure rate was clearly higher in the placebo group than in the group on 2 g/day of acamprosate (68.4% vs. 50.3%; $p=0.01$). In addition, one of the decisive factors in the outcome was the duration of detoxification which was statistically longer in the responders, regardless of the study treatment (20 days±10 vs. 16.8±7.2; $p=0.0005$). This finding is confirmed by a most significantly higher failure rate associated with very short hospital stays of 5–9 days, compared with that of hospital stays of 30 days or more (74.9% vs. 44.4%; $p=0.002$). The failure rate was also higher with patients detoxified as outpatients than with those detoxified in hospital (65% vs. 58%), in the whole population.

Among other criteria, the failure rate was higher in the younger patients (65% in the 25- to 34-year-old group vs. 54.3% in the over 54-year-old group), in patients who did not live with their family (70.3% vs. 56%), and in patients with a high anxiety or depression score. Conversely, other patients tended to present a lower failure rate: 46.8% of failures were observed in patients with a very poor quality of life score (≤3) against 59.5% in subjects with a higher score, and 51.6% of failures were found in patients with a daily consumption of more than 200 g of pure alcohol against 62.7% in those whose consumption was lower. Sex, occupational activity, craving for alcohol at inclusion, total duration of alcoholism, number of previous detoxification periods, and duration of abstinence after the last detoxification period did not influence the outcome.

Safety

Six deaths occurred during the course of the study, two in each group. None of these cases was reported as being causally related to treatment. Four deaths were accidental (three traffic accidents, and one fall), one death was due to a mesenteric infarction, and one haematemesis. Thirty-three patients were withdrawn from the trial due to adverse events. A similar number of patients in each group reported adverse events: 61 in the placebo group, 67 in the group on 1.3 g/day of acamprosate, and 69 in the group on 2 g/day. The adverse event most frequently reported with acamprosate was diarrhoea (41 cases). This effect was dose-dependent: 6 patients with placebo, 14 patients with the 1.3 g low dose acamprosate, and 21 patients with the high dose of 2 g ($p<0.01$). The other events most frequently encountered (pruritus, gastritis, nausea, headaches, dizziness, allergic eruption, and weight gain) were equally distributed among the three groups.

Analysis of the Post-treatment Period

After 18 month follow-up, no statistically significant difference was found between the groups in either the proportion of patients presenting with continuous abstinence since detoxification or the level of alcohol craving. The percentage of abstinent patients at the 18th month visit was statistically higher in the group on 2 g/day of acamprosate than in the placebo group ($p=0.002$) as well as with patients who continued to attend the clinic ($p=0.034$).

Discussion

This study confirms the efficacy of acamprosate in helping to maintain abstinence in weaned alcohol-dependent patients. Although the differences observed on the outcome criteria were not statistically significant at every evaluation, there is a striking convergence of the various results, all pointing in the same direction. Acamprosate was shown to be superior to placebo on abstinence, whatever the criteria assessed: maintenance of continuous abstinence, duration of continuous abstinence, longest period of abstinence or cumulated duration of abstinence. There was dose-effect relationship, the dose of 2 g/day being the most efficient on all outcome criteria, while the results obtained with a dose of 1.3 g/day most often came between those of the placebo and those of the high acamprosate dose. Finally, the safety profile of the treatment was good: only episodes of diarrhoea were more frequently reported with acamprosate, this effect being dose-related. Overall, the risk/benefit ratio for acamprosate is judged to be favourable.

The present study also provides other useful information regarding the optimum use of the product, even if the results should be handled with care due to the small sample size in the sub-groups analyses.

First of all, acamprosate appears to improve significantly patient retention in the study: 52% of patients treated with acamprosate remained in the study after 1 year, compared with 35% in the placebo group. The reasons for this improvement in treatment compliance are not totally clear. Most likely the overall better results with patients treated with acamprosate, particularly regarding their alcohol consumption throughout the trial, play an important role. This effect on patient retention is of importance, since several studies have shown that a longer period of follow-up improves the treatment outcomes (Mackenzie et al. 1987; Moos and Bliss 1978; Ornstein and Cherepon 1985). Moreover, it seems that a relapse – even a severe one – would not lead to treatment withdrawal: statistically, the patients treated with 2 g/day of acamprosate had returned to abstinence or to a controlled consumption by the next visit more frequently than patients on placebo. This fact would be worth evaluating in a larger group of patients followed up for a longer period, in order to confirm the results.

The strong craving for alcohol before treatment initiation diminished to the point that, from the 3rd month onward, less than 10% of patients were still suffering from uncontrolled craving. The craving – always weaker with acamprosate than with placebo – did not differ statistically between the three groups except at the 3rd month. The hypothesis that baseline craving was stronger with the patients who withdrew from the trial was not verified. On the other hand, the prognostic role for later results of persistence of a strong craving at 3 months should be mentioned, particularly the fact that acamprosate significantly reduced craving at 3 months with better results in terms of abstinence, or even of controlled consumption, at the subsequent evaluations.

We also tried to determine whether the profile of the patients lost to follow-up during the trial differed from that of the patients who completed it according to the protocol. The patients lost to follow-up appeared to be younger, lived less often with their families, and more often had a job. The duration of abstinence after their last detoxification period was shorter, and their quality of life seemed to be better. Some of these observations, especially in terms of occupational activity and quality of life, may appear to run counter to set ideas. One may, however, hypothesise that these subjects who appeared overall to have fewer problems than the others might also have been less motivated and, consequently, less inclined to comply with follow-up. Conversely, patients more exposed to family pressures and to existential distress (no job, anxiety, poor quality of life, etc.) were perhaps more prone to abstinence and to comply to the treatment regimen. However, no definitive conclusion can be drawn due to the small number of patients lost to follow-up.

Unfortunately, only a few studies in the literature report data on alcohol-dependent patients lost to follow-up during the course of the treatment. They are rather dated and show that patients who prematurely dropped out of the studies were socially more unstable than those who completed the treatment (Mackenzie et al. 1987; Ruggels et al. 1975). In 1987, Fleming and Lewis demonstrated on a small sample of patients that if the personality status of patients is not discriminant there is nevertheless a strong correlation between the drop-out rate and a low socio-economic status. Rees et al. suggested in 1984 that a patient aware of the severity of his disease is a valuable partner for treatment compliance.

Finally, it is worth noting in this study that the duration of admission to detoxification was a most important pronostic factor, regardless of the treatment programme. Higher age, family life, and low anxiety or depression scores also appeared to be favourable factors. In this study, however, the fact that a low quality of life score and significant daily alcohol consumption are associated with a better result is not necessarily as paradoxical as it may seem since, here again, personal discomfort and family pressure may play a part. On the other hand, subgroups of patients likely to respond better to treatment with acamprosate cannot be identified on the basis of this study.

In the literature, prognostic criteria also tend to be more often linked to the patients' profile than to the treatment programme (Schuckit et al. 1986). Crawford (1976), Gottheil et al. (1992), and Ornstein and Cherepon (1995) raised the hospital duration as a predictive factor, but Rueff et al. (1996) did not confirm this hypothesis in his meta-analysis. A higher age, a stable environment, and the socioeconomic level are more widely accepted as predictive factors (Crawford 1976; Ornstein and Cherepon 1985; Seelye 1979).

Conclusion

Our study confirms the pharmacological efficacy of acamprosate in helping to maintain abstinence in weaned alcohol-dependent patients. Acamprosate opens up new possibilities in the treatment of alcoholism. As an adjunct to psychotherapy, it is a valuable contribution to the integrative management of this multifactorial disease. However, not all patients responded to acamprosate, and further work is needed to identify the profile of those patients who are particularly sensitive to this pharmacotherapy.

Finally, acamprosate - as the first specific treatment for alcohol dependence with no antabuse effect - has the added value of helping patients and doctors to acknowledge alcoholism as a real disease, removing moral considerations and the guilt feeling. Thus, it enhances the efficacy of the management of the disease (Paille 1993).

References

Covi L, Lipman RS (1984) Primary depression or primary anxiety! A possible psychometric approach to a diagnostic dilemma. Clin Neuropharmacol 7 (Suppl 3): 924-925

Crawford RJM (1976) Treatment success in alcoholism. NZ Med J 84: 93-96

Fleming B, Lewis SA (1987) Factors associated with compliance in the follow-up treatment of alcoholism. Alcohol Alcohol 22: 297-300

Gottheil E, McLellan AT, Druley KA (1992) Length of stay, patient severity and treatment outcome: sample data from the field of alcoholism. J Stud Alcohol 53: 69-75

Lehert P (1993) Review and discussion of the statistical analysis of controlled clinical trials in alcoholism. Alcohol Alcohol [Suppl 2]: 157-163

Lhuintre JP, Moore ND, Saligaut C, Boismare F, Daoust M, Chretien P, Tran G, Hillemand B (1985) Ability of calcium bis acetyl homotaurinate, GABA agonist, to prevent relapse in weaned alcoholics. Lancet 1: 1015-1016

Lhuintre JP, Moore ND, Tran G, Steru L, Langrenon S, Daoust M, Parot P, Ladures P, Libert C, Boismare F, Hillemand B (1990) Acamprosate appears to decrease alcohol intake in weaned alcoholics. Alcohol Alcohol 25: 613-622

Mackenzie A, Funderburk FR, Allen RP, Stefan RL (1987) The characteristics of alcoholics frequently lost to follow-up. J Stud Alcohol 48: 119-123

Moos R, Bliss R (1978) Difficulty of follow-up and outcome of alcoholism treatment. J Stud Alcohol 39: 473-490

Ornstein P, Cherepon JA (1985) Demographic variables as predictors of alcoholism treatment outcome. J Stud Alcohol 46: 425-432

Paille F, Bouix JC, Désobry P, Helven R, Lefrançois J, Huriez A, Parot P (1993) Le suivi du patient alcoolique en médecine générale. Une enquête nationale aupès de 2231 généralistes. Rev Prat Med Gen 7: 41-44

Paille F, Guelfi JD, Perkins AC, Royer RJ, Steru L, Parot P (1995) Double-blind randomised multicentre trial of acamprosate in maintaining abstinence from alcohol. Alcohol Alcohol 30: 239-247

Pelc I, Lebon O, Verbanck P, Lehert P, Opsomer L (1992) Calcium acetylhomotaurinate for maintaining abstinence in weaned alcoholic patients: a placebo controlled double-blind multicentre study. In: Naranjo CA, Sellers E (eds) Novel pharmacological interventions in alcoholism, Springer, Berlin Heidelberg New York, pp 348-352

Raskin A, Schilterbrant J, Reatig N, Mackeon JJ (1969) Replication of factors of psychopathology in interview, ward behavior and self-reporting ratings of hospitalized depressives. J Nerv Ment Dis 148: 87-98

Rees DW, Beech HR, Hore BD (1984) Some factors associated with compliance in the treatment of alcoholism. Alcohol Alcohol 19: 303-307

Rueff B, Batel P, Poynard T (1996) Traitement de l'alcoolo-dépendance psychique. Analyse et méta-analyse de 288 études contrôlées. Libbey Eurotexte, Paris (to be published)

Ruggels WL, Armor DJ, Polich JM, Mothershead A, Stephen MA (1975) A follow-up study of clients at selected Alcoholism Treatment Center funded by NIAAA. Final report. Prepared for the National Institute on Alcohol Abuse and Alcoholism, Ment Park, CA, Stanford Research Institute

Schuckit MA, Schwei MG, Gold E (1986) Prediction of outcome in inpatient alcoholics. J Stud Alcohol 47: 151-155

Seelye EE (1979) Relationship of socio-economic status, psychiatric diagnosis and sex on outcome of alcoholism treatment. J Stud Alcohol 40: 57-62

Clinical Efficacy of Acamprosate in the Treatment of Alcoholism

M. Soyka

Introduction

The pathophysiological and neurochemical basis of alcohol dependence, craving, and relapse are not yet fully understood (for review see Littleton et al. and Lovinger, this volume). However, a variety of studies implicate several neurotransmitters and receptors as very likely to be involved in the development of alcohol tolerance and dependence, including the dopaminergic and serotonergic system (DiChiara and Imperato 1988; Engel et al. 1990; LeMarquand et al. 1994: Sellers et al. 1981, 1992), opiates/endorphines, GABA, and glutamate (Littleton et al. 1991; Lovinger et al. 1989). This has led to new pharmacotherapeutic approaches in the therapy of alcoholism. In addition to chemical aversion therapy (Annis and Peachey 1992; Banys 1988; Fuller et al. 1986), tricyclic antidepressants (Soyka and Naber 1992), and lithium (Fawcett et al. 1984), various other substances have been tested in an attempt to increase abstinence rates in alcoholics, all with little or no success. More recently a variety of substances have been examined as an adjunct in relapse prevention in alcoholism; these include serotonergic substances, especially serotonin uptake inhibitors, buspirone, dopaminergic drugs, and opiate antagonists such as naltrexone and nalmefene (Amit et al. 1991; Balldin et al. 1994; Mason et al. 1994; O'Malley et al. 1992; Sellers et al. 1981; Volpicelli et al. 1992; for review see Soyka 1995). None of these compounds has so far found general exceptance as anticraving drug.

In recent years alcohol research has focused on excitatory amino acids such as glutamate in mediating some of the acute reinforcing effects of alcohol (Rassnick et al. 1992) and on a dysfunction of certain glutamate receptor subtypes [specifically *N*-methyl-D-aspartate (NMDA) receptors]. Changes in the glutamatergic neurotransmission are suspected to be responsible for alcohol craving, relapse, and a number of alcohol-related neuropsychiatric disorders such as seizures and Wernicke-Korsakoff syndrome (for review see Tsai et al. 1995). Alcohol itself has been found to inhibit the activity of the NMDA receptor subtype.

Psychiatrische Klinik der Ludwig-Maximilians-Universität, Nußbaumstr. 7, 80336 München, Germany

Acamprosate: Mode of Action

The use of NMDA antagonists for the treatment of alcohol-related disorders has been advocated repeatedly (Tsai et al. 1995). Most in vitro studies have used MK-801 as a noncompetitive NMDA, antagonist but this compound has proven too toxic for clinical use in humans.

A number of preclinical and in vitro studies have focused on the action of the homotaurinate derivative calcium acetylhomotaurinate, acamprosate, on cell membranes (for review see Zieglgänsberger et al., this volume). The pharmacological profile of acamprosate has been the subject of intensive in vitro and in vivo studies for more than a decade. The drug's mechanism of action was initially believed to be mediated via GABA receptors (Boismare et al. 1984), but this has been questioned by more recent findings (Zeise et al. 1993, 1994). Some earlier studies suggested that the drug may interact with noradrenergic and serotoninergic neurotransmission (Daoust et al. 1989), but this too has been questioned by other studies (Boismare et al. 1986). Some findings suggest some opiate antagonist action (LeMagnen et al. 1987), but these findings must yet be replicated. More recently acamprosate was found to reduce CA^{2+} fluxes and the postsynaptic efficacy of excitatory amino acid neurotransmitters such as L-glutamate (especially NMDA subtype), thus lowering the neuronal excitability (Daoust et al. 1987, 1994; Lhuintre et al. 1985; Zeise et al. 1993; Zieglgänsberger and Zeise 1992). Acamprosate is a potent antagonist of excitatory amino acids' stimulatory effect. Animal studies show that the drug crosses the blood-brain barrier. It has proven to be efficient in reducing alcohol intake both in animal models (Boismare et al. 1984; LeMagnen et al. 1987a,b; LeMagnen 1990; Gewiss et al. 1991; LeMagnen 1990) and some initial human trials (Lhuintre et al. 1985, 1990) without changing ethanol toxicity (LeMagnen et al. 1987) and with no evidence for an abuse potential (Grant and Woolverton 1989). Some studies have even found acamprosate to have some anti-acetaldehyde effect and thus to reduce alcohol toxicity (Durlach et al. 1988). The mechanism of action is discussed in detail by Littleton et al. and by Zieglgänsberger et al. (this volume).

Clinical Efficacy

Initial Studies

The initial studies on the efficacy of acamprosate in relapse prevention in alcoholics were conducted in France by Lhuintre et al. (1985, 1990). The initial single center study of 85 patients found a significant reduction in the proportion of relapses within 3 months after cessation of alcohol use. Acamprosate was given at a daily dose of 25 mg/kg body weight. These findings were corroborated by a later study by these authors and by other clinical studies (reviewed by Aubin, this volume). The results of a clinical trial performed by Pelc et al. 1992 are presented in this volume.

Table 1. Acamprosate: clinical studies performed

Study	Country	No. of patients		Study design	
		Acamprosate	Placebo	Treatment period (months)	Follow-up (months)
Phase II					
Paille et al. (1995)	France	361	177	12	6
Pelc et al. (1994)	Belgium, France	126	62	3	-
Phase III					
Barrias et al.(1995)	Portugal	150	152	12	6
Geerlings and Ansoms (1995)	Belgium, Netherlands	128	134	6	6
Besson et al. (1994)	Switzerland	55	55	12	12
Ladewig et al. (1995)	Switzerland	29	32	6	6
Lesch et al. (1994)	Austria	224	224	12	12
Pelc et al. (1992)	Belgium	55	47	6	-
Poldrugo et al. (1994)	Italy	122	124	6	6
Sass et al. (1995)	Germany	136	136	12	12
Tempesta et al. (1995)	Italy	164	166	6	3
Chick et al. (1995)	United Kingdom	289	292	6	1.5
Phase IV					
Aubin et al. (1994)	France	591	-	0.5	-
Total		2430	1601	-	-

Recent Studies

In recent years the efficacy of the drug has been examined in a number of phase II III and IV studies including several large placebo-controlled, double-blind studies in various European countries on more than 4000 patients (Table 1). Length of treatment, number of patients enrolled, concomitant treatment (disulfiram), and principal efficacy criteria varied between studies. The methodology of the various studies is outlined by A.S. Potgieter and P. Lehert (this volume). Two studies examined different doses of acamprosate (1.3 or 2 g/ day; Paille et al. 1995; Pelc et al. 1994; see below), and in one study disulfiram was given (Besson et al. 1994).

The clinical trials reported in this review all followed a core protocol and were carried out in accordance with the guidelines of good clinical practice in Europe. Since only some of these have been published so far, some figures given below relate to unpublished data which must still be examined carefully in more detail. All published data are presented in the reference list.

The primary outcome criteria were: (a) abstinence/relapse/missing assessment at each visit, (b) time to first relapse (survival analysis), and (c) cumulative abstinence duration (a mathematic sum of all abstinent periods as proposed by Lehert 1993).

The following randomized placebo-controlled double-blind (phase III) studies are reviewed in this article:

12 month (48-week) treatment phase
- Sass et al. (1995), Germany
- Barrias et al. (unpublished data), Portugal
- Besson et al. (1994), Switzerland
- Paille et al. (1995), France
- Lesch et al. (1994), Austria (See also Whitworth et al. 1996)

3- or 6-month treatment phase
- Tempesta et al. (1994), Italy
- Poldrugo et al. (1994), Italy
- Geerlings and Ansoms (unpublished data), Belgium, Netherlands, Luxembourg
- Ladewig et al. (1993), Switzerland
- Chick et al. (unpublished data), United Kingdom
- Pelc et al. (1994), Belgium

The abstinence rates, survival analysis, and cumulative abstinence duration (CAD; number of abstinent days during the studies; see A. Potgieter and P. Lehert, this volume) are demonstrated in Figs. 1–3. With the exception of the study conducted in the United Kingdom by Chick and coworkers (1995) all clinical trials show acamprosate to be superior to placebo with respect to abstinence rates.

With respect to the 12-month studies, Barrias et al. (1995) found 39% of patients on acamprosate to be abstinent at the end of treatment compared to 26% of those on placebo ($p < 0.05$, see Fig. 4) while CAD was significantly longer in the verum group (181 vs. 130 days, $p=0.003$). In the Besson et al. (1994) study CAD was 137 days in the acamprosate group and 75 days in the verum group. These data have been confirmed by the other studies, although the abstinence rates differ considerably between studies and were extremely poor for the UK study (Chick et al. 1995). These variations are possibly due to such factors as characteristics of patients included and concomitant psychosocial treatment (see A. Potgieter and P. Lehert, this volume). Chick and colleagues (unpublished data) found only 11.1% of the patients in the acamprosate and 11.3% of those in the placebo group to be abstinent at the end of the 24-week trial. At the end of the study data were available for 35% in the acamprosate and 37% in the placebo group. Some other important studies are discussed in more detail below. Although no meta-analysis of these data has been performed yet, the results of the respective studies, clearly indicate the drug's ability to increase abstinence rates in alcoholics in various clinical settings and countries.

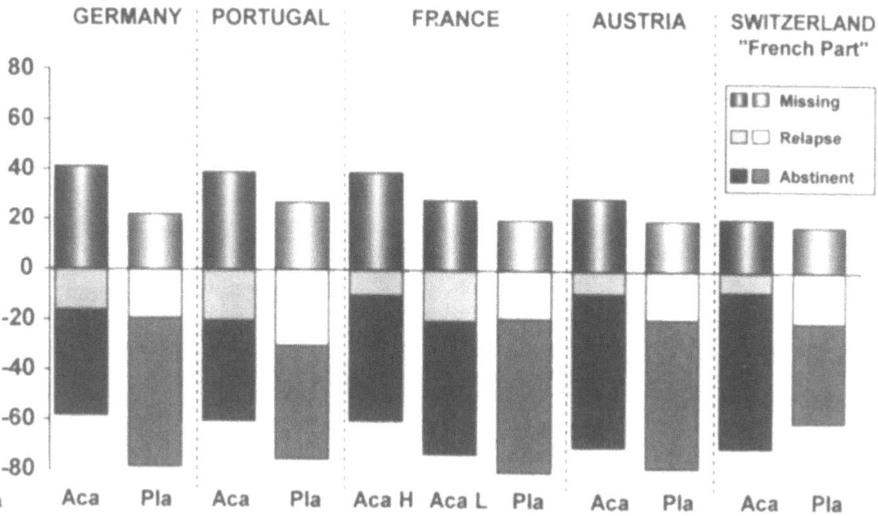

a

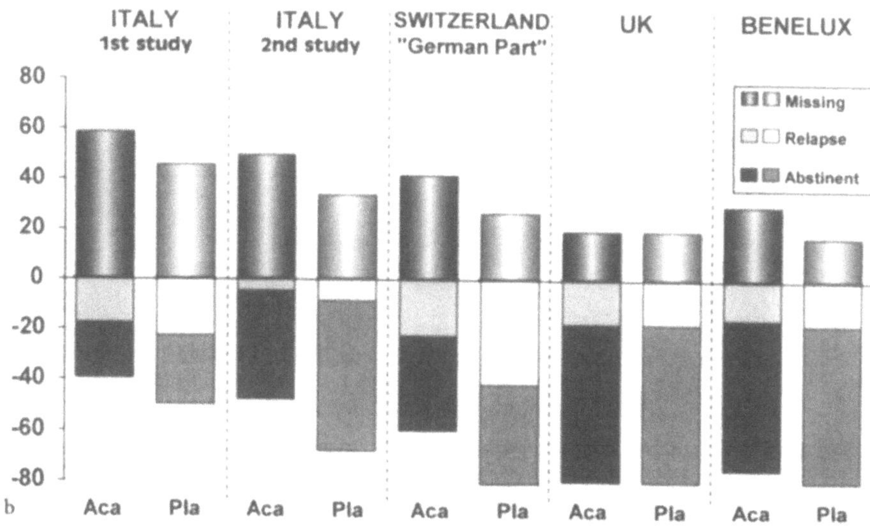

b

Fig. 1a,b. Rates of abstinence, relapse and missing data in studies comparing acamprosate (*Aca*) and Placebo (*Pla*). **a** Studies with 12-month (48-week) treatment phase: Sass et al. (1995). Barrias et al. (1995), Paille et al. (1995), Whitworth et al. (1996), Besson et al. (1994). **b** Studies with 3- or 6-month treatment phase: Tempesta et al. (1995), Poldrugo et al. (1995), Chick et al. (1995), Geerlings and Ansoms (1995)

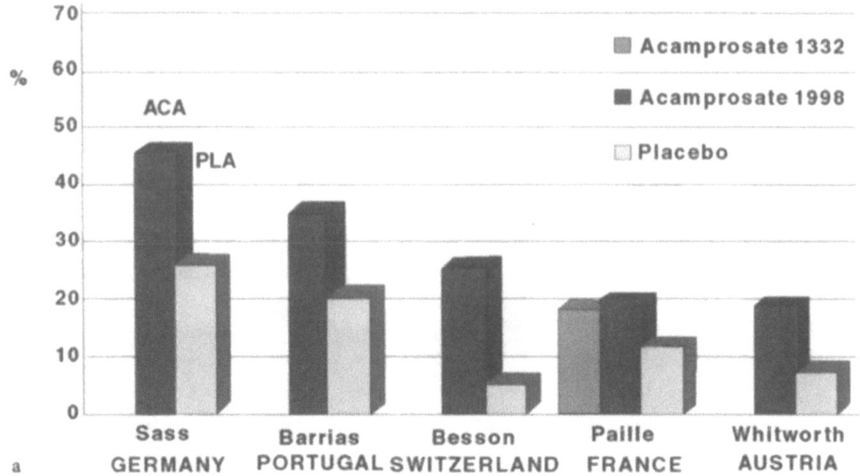

a

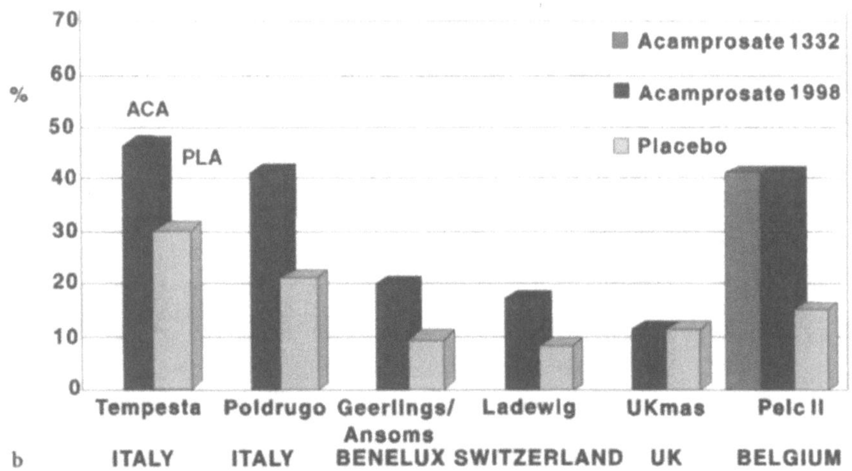

b

Fig. 2a,b. Survival analysis comparing acamprosate (*Aca*) and placebo (*Pla*). **a** Studies with 12-month (48-week) treatment phase: Sass et al. (1995), Barrias et al. (1995), Besson et al. (1994), Paille et al. (1995), Whitworth et al. (1996). **b** Studies with 3- or 6-month treatment phase: Tempesta et al. (1995), Poldrugo et al. (1995), Ladeweig et al. (1995), Chick et al. (1995; *UKmas*), Geerlings and Ansoms (1995), Ladewig et al. (1995), Chick et al. (1995; *UKmas*), Pelc et al. (1994; *Pelc II*)

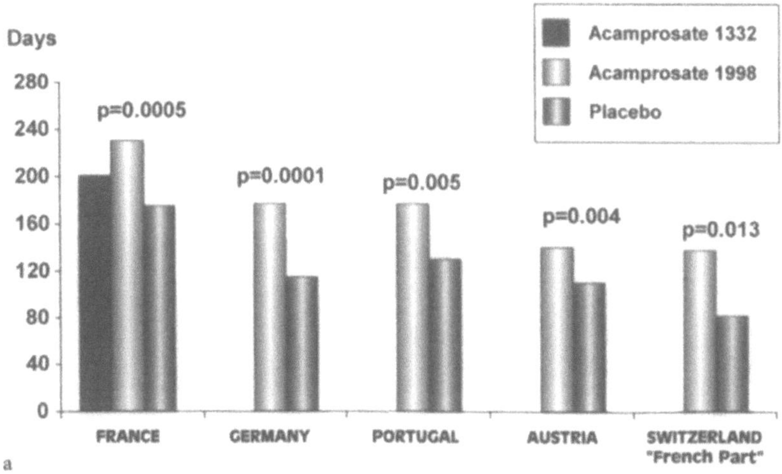

a

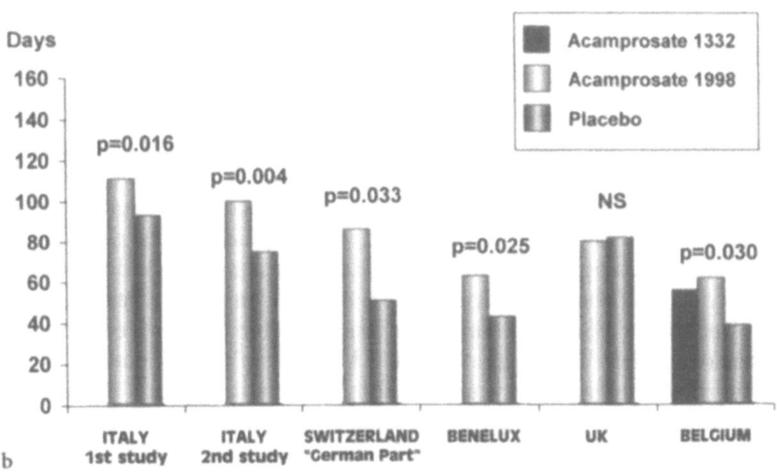

b

Fig. 3a,b. Cumulative abstinence duration in studies comparing acamprosate (*Aca*) and placebo (*Pla*). **a** Studies with 12-months (48-week) treatment phase: Paille et al. (1995), Sass et al. (1995), Barrias et al. (1955), Whitworth et al. (1996), Besson et al. (1994). **b** Studies with 3- or 6-month treatment phase: Tempesta et al. (1995), Poldrugo et al. (1995), Ladewig et al. (1995), Geerlings and Ansoms (1995), Chick et al. (1995; *UKmas*), Pelc et al. (1994; *Pelc II*)

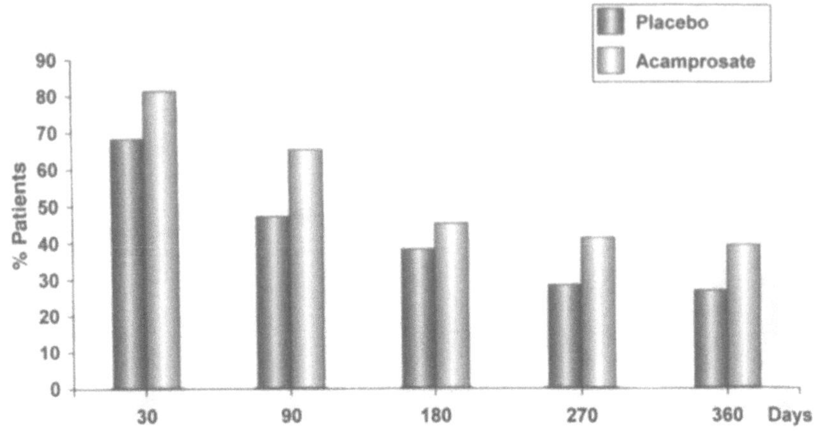

Fig. 4. Percentage of patients abstinent at each evaluation visit. (From Barrias et al. 1995)

The German Study by Sass et al. (1995)

Subjects and Methods

A total of 272 alcoholic patients recruited in 14 collaborating centers took part in a randomized, double-blind, placebo-controlled study (phase III) which consisted of a 48-week treatment phase and a 48-week drug-free follow-up (Sass et al. 1995). Patients were recruited both as in- and outpatients within 4 weeks following alcohol detoxification. The diagnostic process included a careful somatic-neurological examination, a large semistructured interview to establish medical, alcohol, and drug history and demographic variables, the Göttinger Dependence Scale (*Abhängigkeitsskala*) which is derived from the SADQ (Stockwell et al. 1979), the Munich Alcoholism Test (Feuerlein et al. 1977), a neuropsychological test, and various other instruments. Patients included met the criteria for alcohol dependence defined by the third revised edition of the *Diagnostic and Statistical Manual of Mental Disorders.* Patients with severe neuropsychological impairment, neurological or somatic disorders such as liver cirrhosis, epilepsy, and hyperparathyroidism, or polytoxicomania were excluded from the study. The biostatistical analysis showed no relevant baseline inhomogeneities in the distribution of variables such as drinking history between the verum and the placebo groups. Patients received 6×333 mg (body weight ≥ 60 kg) or 4×333 mg acamprosate (< 60 kg) or placebo. the starting dose could be adjusted individually during treatment phase. At several follow-up points during the 48-week trial the patient's drinking status (relapse?) and tolerance of the drug was clinically assessed including regular respiratory alcohol tests. In addition, γ-glutamyltranspeptidase (GGT), glutamic oxaloacetic transaminase, glutamic pyruvic transaminase, macrocytosis (MCV), and carbohydrate deficient (CD)-transferrin were used as objective criteria.

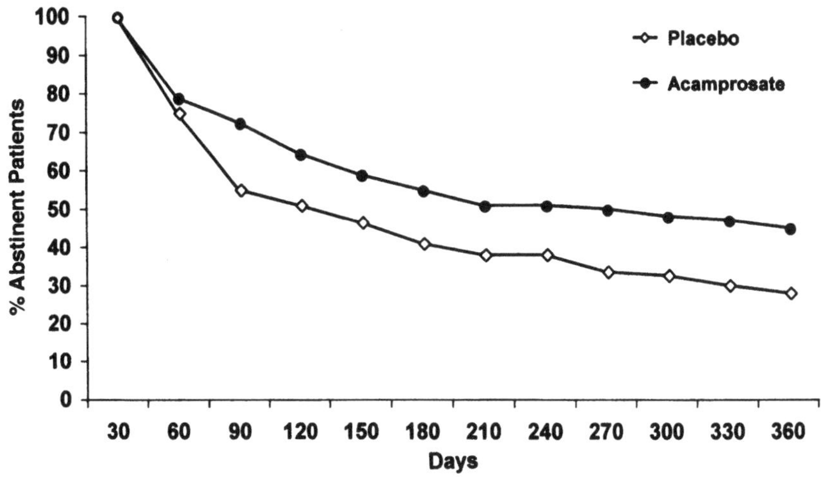

Fig. 5. Time to first relapse. (From Sass et al. 1995)

Results

Of the 272 patients enrolled, 134 (49.3%) completed the study after 1 year. The statistical analysis showed the following:

- Patients on acamprosate showed significantly higher abstinence rates within the first 60 days of treatment (67% vs. 50%) and throughout the further study (45% vs. 25%, see Fig. 5) and had a significantly longer CAD (224 vs. 163 days, or 62% vs. 45% days abstinent; $p < 0.001$). Psychiatric assessments indicated no differences between the two groups. In the acamprosate group 41% of patients had dropped out, compared to 60% in the placebo group.
- GGT values were significantly lower in the acamprosate group throughout and at the end of the study.
- Very few side effects were recorded, mainly diarrhoea and headache. Both acamprosate and placebo were usually well tolerated, and no significant differences were observed with respect to serious adverse reactions.

The French Study by Paille et al. (1995)

In most studies patients weighing more than 60 kg received 2 g acamprosate per day. Few of the studies have addressed the question of whether lower doses might show similar effects. This problem was considered in two studies, those performed by Paille et al. (1995) and by Pelc et al. (1994).

Subjects and Methods

A prospective, placebo-controlled, randomized, double-blind study of acamprosate was performed by Paille et al. (1995) in alcohol-dependent patients who were followed up for 12 months. A total of 538 patients were included in the study and were randomly assigned to a placebo group (n=177) or to one of the two acamprosate groups (1.3 or 2 g/day for 12 months), followed by a single-blind 6-month period or placebo.

Results

Abstinence rates followed the order: high dose > low dose > placebo; significant differences were observed between groups at 6 months ($p < 0.02$) but not at 12 months (p=0.09). The number of days of continuous abstinence after detoxification were 153 ± 189 days (high-dose group) versus 102 ± 165 in the placebo group (p=0.005), with the low-dose group lying between these (135 ± 189 days; see Figs. 6, 7). These findings were corroborated by measurement of biological markers such as GGT. Compliance was highest in the high-dose group, followed by the low-dose group and the placebo group.

No increased relapse rate of residual drug effect was observed during the 6-month post-treatment period. As in other studies, the side effect profile for acamprosate was good compared with controls, with diarrhoea being the only side effect reported more frequently.

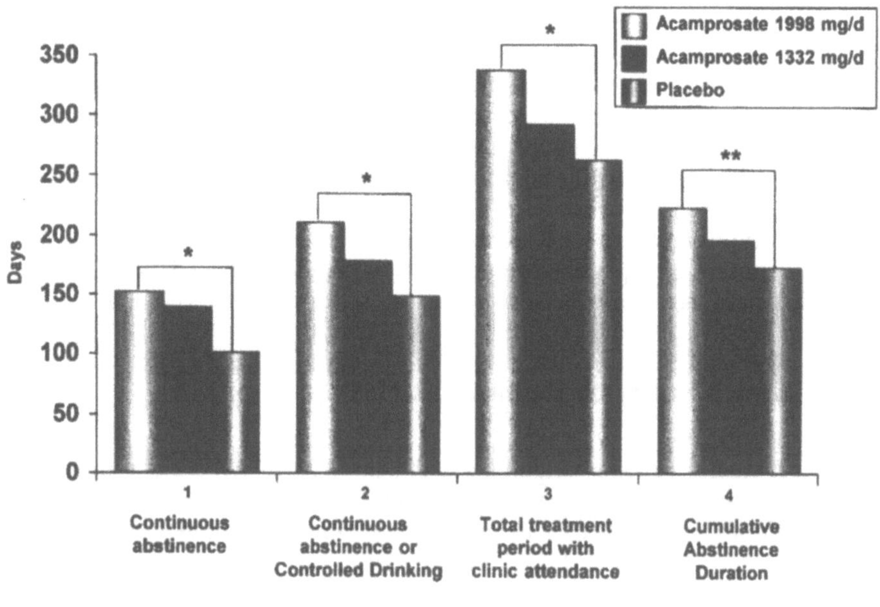

Fig. 6. Results of treatment with two doses of acamprostate in 538 weaned alcoholics. Comparison with placebo on various parameters. *p < 0.01; **p < 0.001. (From Paille et al. 1995)

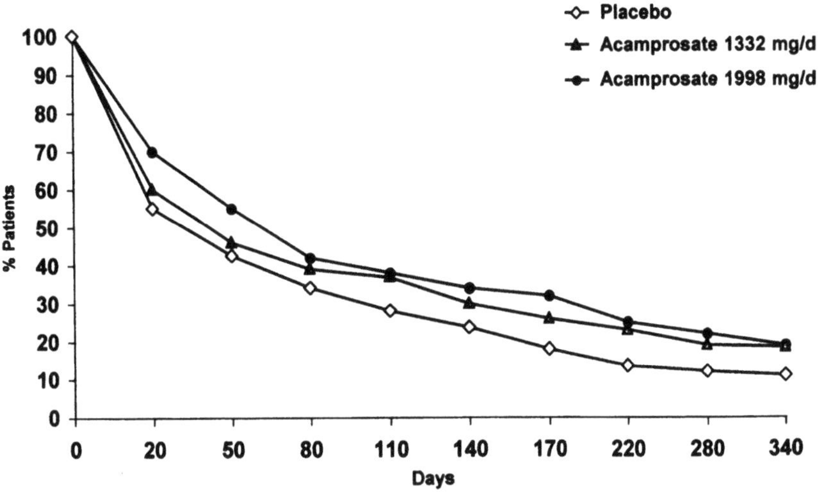

Fig. 7. Percentage of patients with continuous abstinence from alcohol since day 0. (From Paille et al. 1995)

In a similar study performed by Pelc and coworkers (1995; Figs. 8, 9) both dosages of acamprosate (2 or 1.4 g/day) were found to be superior to placebo with respect to abstinence, with no significant differences between the high- and low-dose groups.

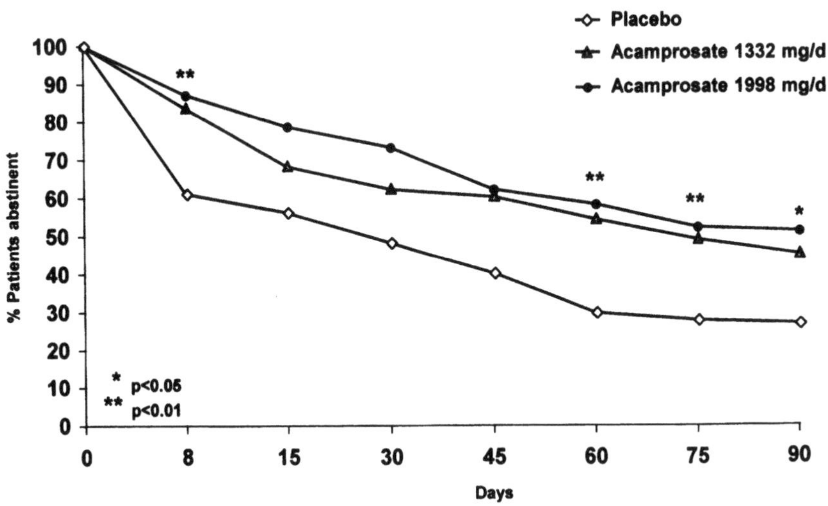

Fig. 8. Percentage of patients abstinent at each evaluation day. (From Pelc et al. 1994)

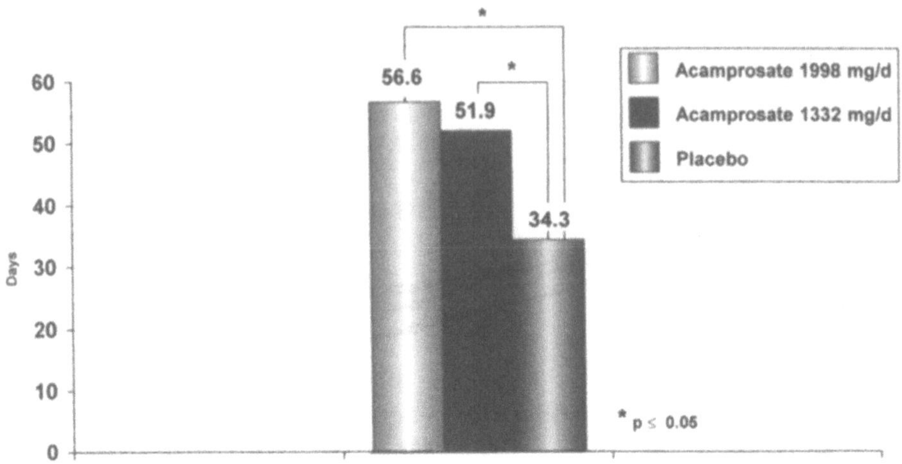

Fig. 9. Cumulative abstinence duration. * $p \leq 0.05$. (From Pelc et al. 1994)

Discussion

With the exception of the study by Chick et al. (1995) all randomized, placebo-controlled clinical studies show higher abstinence rates in patients who received acamprosate than in those who received placebo. Acamprosate was found to reduce relapse rates in recently detoxified alcoholics, as indicated by a higher number of patients in the acamprosate group being abstinent during and at the end of the studies, and a greater number of abstinent days during treatment, as measured by the CAD index (Lehert 1993). In contrast to some studies in the United States (O'Malley et al. 1992; Volpicelli et al. 1992), relapse was defined as *any* alcohol intake. The methodology of clinical trials assessing the ability of a drug to reduce relapse rates in alcoholics is still a matter of controversy (for review see The Plinius Maior Society 1994; Soyka 1995), but the studies cited in this review all followed a core protocol and were conducted according to the European guidelines of good clinical practice.

Some of the methodological and clinical problems concerning pharmacotherapeutic trials in alcoholics and treatment with acamprosate are discussed briefly below.

1. There is an obvious need to develop better instruments and markers for (quantitative) measurement of both alcohol consumption (e.g., biological markers) and the psychopathological and neurobiological basis and consequences of alcoholism. However, in the studies reviewed here, substantial effort was taken to measure alcohol intake adequately and to obtain any possible information on patients who dropped out during the treatment phase or follow-up. The information base included detailed interviews and information from general practioners and family members. Biological markers are less subject to observer variations. Therefore GGT values were measured in all of the studies mentioned. Another biological parameter tested in some of the

studies was carbohydrate deficient transferrin, which has been advocated as the most valid markers in alcoholism. Thus the obtained data for abtinence/relapse may be considered valid.

2. The adequate statistical analysis of pharmacotherapeutic trials in alcoholics must be discussed. In addition to general problems such as measurement of compliance by adequate urine/blood analysis, the expected high drop-out rate during follow-up and the definition of criteria for survival analysis require specific attention. In alcoholism trials the drop-out rate is comparatively high, and these patients are usually expected as failures, even from the beginning of the trial, regardless of a possible improvement during further treatment. Exclusion of these patients from further analysis may constitute bias. Following the guidelines of Lehert (1993), true drop-outs are defined only as patients with serious adverse events, death, protocol violation (e.g., noncompliance, other exclusion criteria), refusal to continue, or drop-out without any knowledge of outcome. The estimated number of abstinent days during treatment was assessed by means of the CAD index. Thus the estimation of efficacy was based on both relapse occurrence during treatment period and assessment of total days of abstinence.

3. The relationship between craving and relapse warrants further attention. Drugs decreasing alcohol intake in alcoholics are often considered to be "anticraving drugs," although the term craving is very controversial in the literature (for review see Pickens and Johanson 1991). The studies reviewed in this paper attempted to measure the intensity of craving by a visual analogue scale which, according to the preliminary data available so far, failed to demonstrate any clear relationship between intensity of craving and later relapse. Other and better diagnostic instruments for the measurement of craving may have shown different results, but the question remains as to whether drugs such as acamprosate should be termed anticraving drugs. The present author prefers the terms antidipsotropics or antidipsotropic agents, which do not imply any specific mechanism of action.

4. The optimal starting point and ideal optimal length of treatment with antidipsotropic agents such as acamprosate require further attention. The most distinct differences between acamprosate and placebo treatment were observed between days 30 and 90. This suggests that the drug is most effective when given in the first months of abstinence, although it proved to be effective during all the various treatment periods. Analysis of the follow-up data available so far indicates that discontinuiation of the drug does not lead to withdrawal symptoms or alcohol relapse, but this sensitive period of treatment needs to be examined in more detail in future studies.

Clinical Conclusions

As in previous studies (Lhuintre et al. 1985, 1990), acamprosate was found to increase abstinence rates in recently detoxified alcoholics and therefore proved to be an efficient agent in relapse prevention. Few side effects and adverse reactions were observed during the studies, with nausea and diarrhea being the most frequent complications (Lesch et al. 1994; Sass et al. 1995). Tolerance was usually good. The toxicity of the drug is related mainly to the calcium part of the molecule; thus patients with hyperparathyroidism should not be treated with acamprosate. There is no evidence of any psychotropic effect of acamprosate that could account for the observed effect on alcohol intake, and there is apparently no abuse potential (Grant and Woolverton 1989) or interaction with ethanol toxicity.

The underlying mechanism of action of acamprosate is still a matter of controversy. Currently it seems that the reduction of nCa^{2+} fluxes and the postsynaptic efficacy of excitatory amino acid neurotransmitters (L-glutamate and others), resulting in a lowering of neuronal excitability (Zieglgänsberger and Zeise 1992; Zeise et al. 1993), are likely mechanisms involved in reducing relapse rates in alcoholics. Opiate receptors and excitatory amino acid neurotransmitters (Lovinger et al. 1989) and voltage-dependent calcium currents (Littleton et al. 1991) have been implicated in the development of alcohol dependence. Together with possible opiate-antagonist action (LeMagnen 1987) and/or interaction with the serotonergic system (see Hegerl et al., this volume), it seems to be the ability to lower neuronal excitability due to a reduction in nCa^{2+} fluxes and to blunt the action of excitatory amino acids that account for the observed effect.

In addition to other pharmacological agents such as serotonin uptake inhibitors, buspirone, and opiate antagonists which must still be examined in a larger number of patients, acamprosate at present seems to be the most promising anticraving, or antidipsotropic, drug - with a very strong data base of over 4000 patients studied so far. A more detailed analysis of the clinical data obtained in the cited studies and further studies on acamprosate may address some of the open questions concerning the drug's effect in and interaction with different treatment settings and populations, possible interactions with other drugs, optimal time of treatment initiation and duration of treatment, and its effect on different subtypes of alcoholics (Lesch et al. 1994; Pelc et al. 1994; Poldrugo et al. 1994). The latter questions play an important role not only for pharmacotherapeutic trials but also for clinical studies in alcoholics in general. With respect to drug interactions it is important that the concomitant use of tetrabamate, meprobamate, or oxazepam, which are frequently used for alcohol detoxification do not increase the incidence of clinical or biological adverse events (Aubin et al. 1994).

Finally, some possible future indications should be mentioned. The pharmacological profile of acamprosate in some animal models (Gutierrez et al. 1987) indicate that acamprosate may be effective in symptoms of alcohol withdrawal. A number of recent preclinical studies suggest that the noncompetitive NMDA antagonist MK-801 blocks the development of tolerance or dependence to several psychoactive substances, including opiates and psychostimulants (Karler et al. 1989; Trujilo and Akil 1991). Since both dopamine and NMDA receptors seem to play an important role in morphine tolerance and dependence (Verma and Kulkarni 1995), NMDA modulators such as acamprosate may be effective in some patients with substance abuse other than alcohol. Finally, since the glutamatergic neurotransmission seems to be of great importance for memory effects and learning (Tsai et al. 1995), NMDA antagonists may be effective in reducing memory deficits in patients with alcoholic amnestic disorder or other organic brain syndromes. None of these speculative hypotheses has been addressed even in pilot studies, but future research may lead to new, unexpected, and exciting new indications for drugs such as acamprosate.

In conclusion, acamprosate and hopefully some other pharmacotherapeutic agents will provide new therapeutic chances for alcoholics and may contribute to a better prognosis and treatment outcome in alcoholics.

References

Amit Z, Smith BR, Gill KG (1991) Serotonin uptake inhibitors: effects on motivated consummatory behaviors. J Clin Psychiatry 52 [suppl 12]: 55-60

Annis HM, Peachey JE (1992) The use of calcium carbimide in relapse prevention counselling: results of a randomized controlled trial. Br J Addict 87: 63-72

Aubin HJ, Lehert P, Beaupere B, Jacquemin F, Barrucand D (1994) Acamprosate tolerance in association with other medications taken during alcohol withdrawal. Multicentre trial involving 591 alcoholic patients undergoing withdrawal. Alcoologie 16: 32-41

Balldin J, Berggren U, Bokström K, Erikkson M, Gottfries CG, Karlsson I, Walinder J (1994) Six-month open trial with zimelidine in alcohol-dependent patients: reduction in days of alcohol intake. Drug Alcohol Depend 35: 245-248

Banys P (1988) The clinical use of disulfiram (Antabuse): review. J Psychoact Drugs 20: 243-261

Besson J, Aeby F, Kasas A, Fendl A, Lehert P (1994) Combined efficacy of acamprosate and disulfiram for enhancing abstinence of chronic alcoholic pateints during a one year post detofixication period. Neuropsychopharmacology 10.3 [Suppl 2]: 74S

Boismare F, Daoust M, Moore N, Saligaut C, Lhuintre JP, Chretien P, Durlach J (1984) A homotaurine derivate reduces the voluntary intake by rats: are cerebral GABA receptors involved? Pharmacol Biochem Behav 21: 787-789

Boismare F, Daoust M, Lhuintre JP, Moore N, Saligaut C, Chretien P (1986) Metaprime-induced reduction of voluntary intake of ethanol by rats: mechanism of action. J Pharmacol 17: 170

Bruno F (1989) Buspirone in the treatment of alcoholic patients. Psychopathology 22 [suppl 1] 49-59

Daoust M, Lhuintre JP, Saligaut C, Moore N, Flipo JL, Boismare F (1987) Noraderenaline and GABA brain receptors are co-involved in the voluntary intake of ethanol by rats. Alcohol Alcohol [suppl]1: 319-322

Daoust M, Protais P, Boucly P, Tran G, Rinjard P, Dokhan R, Fillion G (1989) Intervention of acamprosate on serotoninergic and noradrenergic system. Alcohol Alcohol 24: 370

Daoust M, Legrand E, Durbin P (1994) Binding characteristics of $_3$H-acamprosate on neuronal membrane preparations. Alcohol Clin Exp Res 18: 33A (abstract no 5.13)

DiChiara G, Imperato A (1988) Drugs abused by humans preferentially increase synaptic dopamine concentrations in the mesolimbic system of freely moving rats. Proc Natl Acad Sci USA 85: 5274-5278

Durlach J, Rinjard P, Sprince H, Smith GG (1988) Similar antagonist effects of Ca N-acetyl homotaurinate on depression of motor activity and lethality induced by acetaldehyde or ethanol. Methods Find Exp Clin Pharmacol 10: 437-447

Engel JA, Enerback C, Fahlke C, Hulthe H, Johannenssen K, Stevensson L, Soderpalm B (1990) Serotonergic and dopaminergic involvement in ethanol intake. In: Novel pharmacological interventions for alcoholism. Naranjo CA, Sellers EM (eds) Springer, New York Berlin Heidelberg, pp 68-82

Fawcett J, Clark DC, Gibbons RD, Aagesen CA, Pisani VD, Tilkin JM, Sellers D, Stutzman D (1984) Evaluation of lithium therapy for alcoholism. J Clin Psychiatry 45: 494-499

Feuerlein W, Ringer C, Kuefner H, Antons K (1977) Diagnose des Alkoholismus. Der Münchner Alkoholismustest (MALT). Munch Med Wochenschr 119: 1275-1282

Fuller RK, Branchey L, Brightwell DR, Derman RM, Emrick CD, Iber FL, James KE, Lacoursiere RB, Lee KK, Lowenstamm I, Manny I, Neiderhiser D, Nocks S, Shaw JJ (1986) Disulfiram treatment of alcoholism: a Veterans Aministration cooperative study. JAMA 256: 1449–1455

Gewiss M, Heidbreder C, Opsomer L, Durbin P, De Witte P (1991) Acamprosate and diazepam differentially modulate alcohol induced behavioral and cortical alterations in rats following chronic inhalation of ethanol vapour. Alcohol Alcohol 26: 129–137

Grant KA, Woolverton WL (1989) Reinforcing and discriminative stimulus effects of Ca-acetyl homotraurine in animals. Pharmacol Biochem Behav 32: 607–611

Gutierrez S, Daoust M, Rinjard P, Lhuintre JP, Boismare F (1987) L'acétylhomotaurinate de calcium, molécule a propriétés GABAergiques, atténue le syndrome de sevrage alcoolique chez la souris C57BL. Rev Alcool 32: 241–247

Karler LD, Calder LD, Chaudry IA, Turkanis SA (1989) Blockade of 'reverse tolerance' to cocaine and amphetamine by MK-801. Life Sci 45: 599–606

Ladewig D, Knecht T, Lehert P et al. (1993) Acamprosat – ein stabilisierungstfaktor in der Langzeitentwöhnung von Alkoholabhangigen. Ther Umschau 59: 182–188

Le Magnen J (1990) Effect of calcium acetyl homotaurinate on alcohol dependency. Med Chir Dig 19: 47–48

Le Magnen J, Tran G, Durlach J, Martin C (1987b) Dose-dependent suppression of the high alcohol intake of chronically intoxicated rats by Ca-acetyl homotaurinate. Alcohol 4: 97–102

Lehert P (1993) Review and discussion of statistical analysis of controlled clinical trials in alcoholism. Alcohol Alcohol [Suppl]2: 157–163

LeMarquand D, Pihl RO, Benkelfat C (1994) Serotonin and alcohol intake, abuse, and dependence; clinical evidence. Biol Psychiatry 36: 326–337

Lesch OM, Walter H, Fischer F, Platz W, Haring C, Leitner A, Benda N (1994) New developments of reducing alcohol intake. Alcohol Clin Exp Res 18: 43A (abstract No. 9.3)

Lhuintre JP, Daoust M, Moore N, Cheretien P, Saligaut C, Tran G, Boismare F, Hillemand B (1985) Ability of calcium bis-acetyl homotaurine, a GABA agonsit, to prevent relapse in weaned alcoholics. Lancet I: 1014–1016

Littleton JM, Brennan C, Bouchenafa O (1991) The role of calcium flux in the central nervous system actions of ethanol. Ann N Y Acad Sci 625: 388

Lovinger DM, White G, Weight FF (1989) Ethanol inhibits NMDA-activated ion current in hippocampal neurons. Science 243: 1721

Mason BJ, Ritvo EC, Morgan RO, Salvato FR, Goldberg G, Welch B, Mantero-Atienza E (1994) A double-blind, placebo-controlled pilot study to evaluate the efficacy ans safety of oral nalmefene HCl for alcohol dependence. Alcohol Clin Exp Res 18: 1162–1167

O'Malley SS, Jaffe AJ, Chang G, Schottenfeld RS, Meyer RE, Rounsaville B (1992) Naltrexone and coping skills therapy for alcohol dependence. A controlled study. Arch Gen Psychiatry 49: 881–887

Paille FM, Guelfi JD, Perkins AC, Royer RJ, Steru L, Parot P (1995) Double-blind randomized multicentre trial of acamprosate in maintaining abstinence from alcohol. Alcohol Alcohol 30: 239–247

Pelc I, Lebon O, Verbanck P, Lehert P, Opsomer L (1992) Calcium-acetylhomotaurinate for maintaining abstinence in weaned alcoholic patients: a placebo-controlled double-blind multicenter study. In: Naranjo CA, Sellers EM (eds) Novel pharmacological interventions in alcoholism. Springer, Berlin Heidelberg New York, pp 358–352

Pelc I, LeBon O, Verbanck P (1994) Acamprosate in the treatment of alcohol dependence: a six month post-detoxification study. Alcohol Clin Exp Res 18: 38A (abstract no 6.6)

Pickens RW, Johanson C-E (1991) Craving: consensus of status and agenda for future research. Drug Alcohol Depend 30: 127–131

Poldrugo F, Chabac S, Lehert P (1994) Acamprosate in the long-term treatment of alcoholism: is its use recommended within the psycho-social approach? Alcohol Clin Exp Res 18: 43A (abstract no 9.2)

Rassnick S, Damico E, Riley E, Pulvierenti L, Zieglgänsberger W, Koob GF (1992) GABA and nucleus accumbens glutamate neurotransmission modulate ethanol self-administration in rats. Ann NY Acad Sci 654: 502–555

Sass H, Soyka M, Mann K, Zieglgänsberger W (1995) Relapse prevention by acamprosate: results from a placebo controlled study in alcohol dependence. Arch Gen Psychiatry (in press)

Sellers EM, Naranjo CA, Peachey JE (1981) Drugs to decrease alcohol consumption. N Engl J Med 305: 1255–1262

Sellers EM, Higgins GA, Sobell MB (1992) 5-HT and alcohol abuse. Trends Pharmacol Sci 13: 69–75
Soyka M (1995) Die Alkoholkrankheit. Chapman and Hall, Weinheim
Soyka M, Naber D (1993) Antidepressiva in der Behandlung des chronischen Alkoholismus. Neurol Psychiatr 7: 213–221
Stockwell T, Hodgson R, Edwards G, Taylor C, Rankin H (1979) The development of a questionnaire to measure severity of alcohol dependence. Br J Addict 74: 79–87
Tempesta E, Janiri L, Bignamini A (1994) The effectiveness and safety of calcium-acetylhomotaurinate (acamprosate) on the maintenance and abstinence in weaned alcoholics. Paper given at the 7th AEP congress, 18–22 September 1994, Copenhagen
The Plinius Maior Society (1994) Guidelines on evaluation of treatment of alcohol dependence. Alcoholism 30 [suppl]
Trujillo KA, Akil H (1991) Inhibition of morphine tolerance and dependence by the NMDA receptor antagonist MK-801. Science 251: 85–87
Tsai G, Gastfriend DR, Coyle JT (1995) The glutamatergic basis of human alcoholism. Am J Psychiatry 152: 332–340
Verma A, Kulkarni SK (1993) Role of D_1/D_2 dopamine and N-methyl-D-aspartate (NMDA) receptors in morphine tolerance and dependence in mice. Eur Neupsychopharmacol 5: 81–87
Vollpicelli JR, Alterman AI, Hayashida M, O'Brien CP (1992) Naltrexone in the treatment of alcohol dependence. Arch Gen Psychiatry 49: 876–880
Whitworth AB, Fischer F, Lesch OM, Nimmerrichter A, Oberbauer H, Platz T, Potgieter A, Walter H, Fleischhacker C (1996) Acamprosate versus placebo in the long-term treatment of patients with alcohol dependence. Lancet (in press)
Zeise ML, Kasparow S, Capogna M, Zieglgänsberger W (1993) Acamprosate (calciumhomotaurinate) decreases postsynaptic potentials in the rat neocortex: possible involvement of excitatory amino acid receptors. Eur J Pharmacol 231: 47–52
Zeise ML, Madamba SG, Siggins GR, Putzke J, Zieglgänsberger W (1994) The anti-craving substance acamprosate reduces glutamatergic synaptic transmission and a high-treshold calcium current in neocortical and hippocampal pyramidal neurons. Alcohol Clin Exp Res 18: 36A (abtract no 5.33)
Zielglgänsberger W, Zeise M (1992) Calcium-diacetyl-homotaurinate which prevents relapse in weaned alcoholics decreases the action of excitatory amino acids in neocortical neurons of the rat in vitro. In: Sellers EM, Naranjo CA (eds) Novel pharmacological interventions for alcoholism. Springer, Berlin Heidelberg New York, pp 337–341

Subject Index

Springer-Verlag and the Environment

We at Springer-Verlag firmly believe that an international science publisher has a special obligation to the environment, and our corporate policies consistently reflect this conviction.

We also expect our business partners – paper mills, printers, packaging manufacturers, etc. – to commit themselves to using environmentally friendly materials and production processes.

The paper in this book is made from low- or no-chlorine pulp and is acid free, in conformance with international standards for paper permanency.

MIX
Papier aus verantwortungsvollen Quellen
Paper from responsible sources
FSC® C105338

If you have any concerns about our products,
you can contact us on
ProductSafety@springernature.com

In case Publisher is established outside the EU,
the EU authorized representative is:
Springer Nature Customer Service Center GmbH
Europaplatz 3, 69115 Heidelberg, Germany

Printed by Libri Plureos GmbH
in Hamburg, Germany